PTSD WORKB[...]

OVERCOMING YOUR GREATEST FEARS

A Fun & Light-Hearted Guide To Overcoming Post-Traumatic Stress Disorder For PTSD Recovery

DAMON KENT

The following book is produced below with the goal of providing information that is as accurate and reliable as possible. Regardless, purchasing this eBook can be seen as consent to the fact that both the publisher and the author of this book are in no way experts on the topics discussed within and that any recommendations or suggestions that are made herein are for entertainment purposes only. Professionals should be consulted as needed prior to undertaking any of the action endorsed herein.

This declaration is deemed fair and valid by both the American Bar Association and the Committee of Publishers Association and is legally binding throughout the United States.

Furthermore, the transmission, duplication or reproduction of any of the following work including specific information will be considered an illegal act irrespective of if it is done electronically or in print. This extends to creating a secondary or tertiary copy of the work or a recorded copy and is only allowed with express written consent

Table of Contents

PART I 13

Chapter 1: 14

Understanding Panic Attacks and Panic Disorders 14

What Is a Panic Attack? 15

Anxiety and Panic Attacks Aren't the Same 19

Chapter 3: Biological and Psychological Causes of Panic Attacks 22

Biological Causes of Panic Attacks 22

Psychological Causes of Panic Attacks 25

Chapter 4: Who Is At a Greater Risk of Panic Attacks? 27

Chapter 5: Tips to Cope With Panic Attacks When They Strike 29

Ways to Prevent Panic Attacks 30

Chapter 6: The 8-week Plan to Deal With Panic Attacks 35

Identify the Triggers, Fears, and Problematic Behavior 35

Identify Your Negative Thought Patterns 37

Dissociate From the Negative Thought Patterns 39

Facing the Fears Head-on 41

Practice Relaxation 41

Practice Mindfulness 43

Getting the Experience 44

PART II 45

Chapter 1: Anxiety, The Monster Within 46

How Anxiety Overshadows Everyday Lives 48

What is Anxiety? 49

Causes of Anxiety 50

Signs & Symptoms of Anxiety Disorders 51

Understanding Social Anxiety... 52

Symptoms of Social Anxiety 52

Chapter 2: Acknowledging Your Anxiety...............................55

Common Anxiety Triggers 55

Getting to the Root Causes of Your Anxiety....................... 56

Negative Self-Talk 56

Unrealistic Expectations.. 57

The "Should" Thoughts 57

Taking Things Too Personally 57

Pinpointing Your Anxiety... 58

Chapter 3: Trauma and Anxiety...60

Childhood Trauma and Sensitivity to Anxiety 61

Common Anxiety Disorders Caused by Trauma 61

Chapter 4: Grabbing your life back from anxiety...................63

Managing Your Emotions 63

Don't react right away 63

Find healthy outlets 64

Look at the bigger picture 64

Replace your thoughts 64

Forgive your triggers... 65

Using the Power of Mini Habits.. 65

What Are Mini Habits?... 66

What is *More* Essential than Your *Habits*?...................... 66

Benefits of Mini Habits.. 67

Chapter 5: Belittle anxiety with personal empowerment.......68

Smile.. 68

Focus on solutions, not problems.. 69

Notice the rise, not just the downfall 69

Just breathe 69

Fend off other's negativity 70

Switch the *"I have to"* mindset with *"I get to"* 70

Describe your life positively 71

Master rejection 71

Rethink challenges.. 72

Write in a gratitude journal... 72

Chapter 6: Everyday techniques to fend off anxiety 73

Visualization and Anxiety 73

Why You Should Be Using Visualization............................... 74

Aspects of Successful Visualization Practices...................... 77

Forms of Visualization for Anxiety....................................... 78

Meditation.. 78

Altered Memory Visualization... 79

Receptive Visualization 80

Treasure Map 81

How to Design Your Own "Safe Space"................................. 81

Developing Anxiety Routines 84

Routines to Decrease Anxiety 85

The Importance of a Balanced Morning Routine 86

Benefits of a Morning Routine 87

Steps to Include in Your Morning Routine 87

Other Morning Methods to Relieve Anxiety 90

Chapter 7: Transforming Your anxiety for a better life 91

Using Anxiety to Your Advantage 92

Redefining danger 92

Channel your stress properly 92

Stop trying to do your best 93

Chapter 8: Battling anxiety like a true warrior 94

Spend time preparing 94

Learn to *manage* fear 94

Breathe 95

Don't keep things bottled up 97

Overpower that inner nagging voice 97

Think of the worst-case scenario 98

Reframe your mindset 98

Neuroplasticity 99

Get moving 100

Chapter 9: Rediscovering yourself after hurricane anxiety 102

When were you the *happiest*? 102

What makes you *unhappy*? 102

Write! 103

Learning to Love Yourself Again 103

Care about yourself as much as you care about others 104

Maintain boundaries 104

Do YOU? 106

Chapter 1: Self-Care Is the Best Care 108

How Does Self-Care Work 109

How Does Self-Care Improve Self-Esteem and Self-Confidence? 110

Chapter 2: 113

What Does Good Self-Care Look Like? 113

Good Self-Care Practices.. 113

Taking Responsibility for Your Happiness...................... 113

You Become Assertive With Others.............................. 113

You Treat Yourself As You Would a Close Friend.............. 113

You Are Not Afraid to Ask for What You Want.............. 114

Your Life Is Set Around Your Own Values 114

Chapter 3: Demanding Your Own Self-Care......................... 115

Setting Healthy Boundaries.. 115

Identify and Name Your Limits 115

Stay Tuned Into Your Feelings 116

Don't Be Afraid of Being Direct................................ 116

Give Yourself Permission to Set Boundaries.................. 116

Consider Your Past and Present................................ 117

Be Assertive... 117

Start Small 117

Eliminating Toxicity and Not Caring About Losing Friends................. 118

Don't Expect People to Change................................ 118

Establish and Maintain Boundaries 118

Don't Keep Falling for Crisis Situations 118

Focus on the Solution 119

Accept Your Own Difficulties and Weaknesses 119

They Won't Go Easily.. 119

Choose Your Battles Carefully 120

Surround Yourself With Healthy relationships 120

How to Focus on Self-Care 120

Pay Attention to Your Sleep 120

Take Care of Your Gut 121

Exercise and Physical Activity Is Essential.................................... 121

Consider a Mediterranean Diet 121

Take a Self-Care Trip 122

Get Outside.. 122

Bring a Pet Into Your Life.. 122

Get Yourself Organized 122

Cook Yourself Meals At Home.. 122

Read Regularly... 123

Schedule Your Self-Care Time 123

Chapter 4: How to Be Happy Being Alone.............................. 124

Accept Some Alone Time 124

Do Not Compare Yourself to Others... 124

Step Away From Social Media 124

Take a Break From Your Phone 125

Allow Time for Your Mind to Wander 125

Take Yourself on a Date.. 125

Exercise.. 125

Take Advantage of the Perks of Being Alone................................. 125

Find a Creative Outlet 126

Take Time to Self-Reflect.. 126

Make Plans for Your Future 126

Make Plans for Solo Outings 126

Chapter 1: What is CBT?... 129

The Science Behind It.. 130

How it Works 133

Changes Thought Patterns and Belief Systems 135

Its Purpose – Who it Can Help.. 136

How it Works on Anxiety and Depression.. 138

Depressive Disorders 144

How CBT Helps With Substance Abuse... 146

Chapter 2: How CBT Can Help With… 149

Problem-Solving With Depression or Anxiety 150

CBT with Sleep Disorders 152

Chapter 3: Common Causes of Mood Disorders 155

Chemical Imbalances 156

Chapter 4: Understanding Your Moods and the Way You Think 161

How to Diagnose Your Negative Thought Patterns.......................... 162

Intrusive Thoughts 166

Examples of Some Intrusive Thoughts... 166

Identifying Your Triggers for Anxiety and Stress 168

Chapter 5: How it Treats Mood Disorders 174

Practical Applications of CBT... 174

Setting Goals... 177

Building Self-Esteem 178

Verbal Self-Talk... 180

Counter Negative and Angry Feelings... 181

Dealing With Feelings of Guilt 181

Counteract Hopelessness.. 182

Chapter 6: Steps to Dealing with Mood Disorders and Depression ... 184

Chapter 7: Multimodal Model...188

The Seven Modalities You Should Know About.................................. 189

Chapter 8: Rational Emotive Behavioral Therapy 193

A: Activating Event.. 194

B: The Belief.. 194

C: Consequences.. 194

D: Dispute 194

E: Effect 195

Chapter 9: Dialectical Behavior Therapy 196

PART I

Chapter 1:

Understanding Panic Attacks and Panic Disorders

Imagine the fear of watching a giant wave coming roaring towards you, while you stand frozen, unable to move an inch.

It is frightening. Have you ever experienced any such fear?
Imagine having extreme breathing difficulty all of a sudden, like having an asthma attack, without suffering from asthma.

It's scary and suffocating. Have you been in any such situation ever?
Imagine being in a situation when you are quite sure that you are not going to survive that crisis; only there is no such crisis.

It is a terrible experience. Have you been through it?
These are real-life situations that a panic attack might look like. To an onlooker, a panic may look like an overreaction. Most people consider panic attacks as dodging tactics using which you can escape facing tough situations. However, they are unable to understand that during a panic attack, the victim experiences difficulty in breathing, the actual feeling of an allergic reaction is there.

For many victims, there is a feeling of the throat closing up, feels like throat tightening, and it seems like a reaction of a body as if you were about to die, nausea, heart palpitation, excessive sweating, blackouts, chest pain, and complete loss of control are some of the common symptoms panic attack victims may experience during the attacks.

Panic attacks can come out of the blue without a prior warning or even without triggers. They are scarier than they sound because the panic attack victim can feel them approaching because there's nowhere to run. The warning signal is coming from the inside, and you can't run away from yourself.

Many people start saying breathe deeply, relax, or be calm, but all these suggestions are useless because the words don't reach the effective areas. Deep breathing can help the victim relax and avoid panic attacks, but that advice and assurance must come from inside. The realization that you can avert the attack by simply diverting your mind and staying calm must be there in you. There is no doubt that a panic attack victim would have to work on developing this confidence and realization, but it is very much possible.

What Is a Panic Attack?

Excessive anxieties and fears can lead to panic attacks. During a panic attack, the victim can experience several symptoms like racing heart, heart palpitation, excessive shaking, breathing difficulties, and nausea. Things simply start slipping out of control, and the victim starts feeling very helpless and vulnerable. Every panic attack victim doesn't experience all the symptoms mentioned above. As per the Diagnostic and Statistical Manual of Mental Disorders, fourth edition, if a victim experiences any of the four symptoms from the list given below, the victim is considered to have experienced a panic attack.

The real tell-tale sign of a panic attack is that it builds up rapidly. A person could be doing fine just a few minutes ago, and all of a sudden can start exhibiting signs of fear, anxiety, pain, and discomfort. A panic attack generally reaches its peak within ten minutes of the beginning.

Important Symptoms, the Victim of a Panic Attack, Is Likely to Experience:

(A person experiencing at least four of the symptoms at the same time is classified as experiencing a panic attack.)

1. Sensations of shortness of breath or smothering
2. Palpitations, pounding heart, or accelerated rate of heart
3. Trembling or shaking
4. Feeling lightheaded, unsteady, dizzy, or faint
5. Fear of losing control or going crazy
6. Chills or hot flushes
7. Sweating
8. Feeling of choking
9. Discomfort or chest pain
10. Nausea or abdominal distress
11. Fear of dying
12. Paresthesias (tingling sensations or numbness)
13. Derealization (a sense of unreality) or depersonalization (feeling detached from oneself)

As mentioned above, panic attacks symptoms appear very fast and do not allow the victim to understand much. It can peak within a short span of just 10 minutes, and hence initially, the victims generally do not get a chance to react properly.

A panic attack can make the victim feel like he/she isn't going to survive it. To some, the acute chest pain looks like a heart attack, and to others, the breathing difficulty episodes brought by panic attacks resemble asthma attacks. Most victims end up in emergency rooms only to be told later on that they had a panic attack.

It is important to understand that panic attacks don't last very long. A panic attack can begin out of the blue without a trigger and may reach its peak within 10 minutes. However, in most cases, panic attacks get resolved within half an hour. It is rare for a panic attack to last an hour.

Although panic attacks may last only for half an hour, for the victim, this duration may seem like an eternity. The whole period is physically and emotionally very stressful and overwhelming. It is the extreme stress experienced during the panic attack that may make it feel like a very long period, and it can be emotionally churning.

It is very important to note that there is no specific cause of panic attacks. Panic attacks can be caused by various stressors, and the genetic buildup of a person can make a person prone to panic attacks. However, people with mood disorders and long-standing anxiety issues are naturally soft-targets of panic attacks. Severe stress, major transitions in life, a feeling of acute vulnerability, and several medical conditions can also make a person prone to panic attacks.

What Is Panic Disorder and Should You Be Worried About It?

Panic disorder is having an extended fear of panic attacks all the time, even when you haven't had a panic attack in a month or more.

It is very much possible for a person to just have one or two episodes of panic attacks and then never have them ever. You were passing through a bad patch in life that made you insecure and vulnerable and caused a panic attack. When then phase passes away, you might not experience a panic attack ever again. Unfortunately, some people experience repeated panic attacks, and they undergo substantial behavioral changes making anxiety a part of their lives. They are always anxious about the next attack to come. Such people can be termed as suffering from **Panic Disorder**.

Symptoms That a Person Might be Developing Panic Disorder are:

- Constant worry about panic attacks
- Frequent episodes of panic attacks out of the blue
- Clear avoidance of things and situations that might have led to a panic attack

Panic disorders are the quiet periods between panic attacks, and they can be more harmful than panic attacks as they can severely affect the life and functioning of the victim. They can be as threatening as the silence before a storm, and that's what keeps the victims on edge.

Emotionally, panic disorder can take a toll on the mental health of the victim as it keeps the mind full of fearful thoughts and anxieties. Finding a diversion can get difficult in such a condition. The victims are unable to push the fear of an attack from their mind, and they are always in fear of an impending attack

Chapter 2

Anxiety and Panic Attacks Aren't the Same

There are many common symptoms in anxiety and panic attacks, and that makes people draw a misleading conclusion that having anxiety disorders and panic attacks or panic disorders is all the same.

Very Important

You must make it very clear in your mind that having a panic attack is an easily treatable condition. If you've just had a few episodes of panic attacks, you can just go to a doctor and get treatment for that. A simple medication routine of a fortnight can help you get over panic attacks. However, treatment of anxiety disorders is a very lengthy process that may take years while using both medication and therapy.

Therefore, if you or someone you know just had a panic attack, there is no reason to worry as it is a treatable condition.

Differentiating between both the conditions can be a bit tricky and may need professional help.

However, here are some broad points that can help you understand the difference:

- Anxieties are generally very specific. There are triggers for anxiety. You know the things that can make you feel anxious. There would be specific stressors and triggers that can trigger anxiety in you. On the other hand, panic attacks usually come without a trigger.

- A big difference between anxiety and panic is the way you feel them. Panic attacks are sudden and intense. A panic attack can start all of a sudden without a trigger and would reach its peak in a short span of 10 minutes. Although they are fast and intense and the entire duration of a panic attack may seem like an eternity, usually they don't last longer than half an hour and would rarely extend for an hour. Whereas anxiety can keep building for months.

- Initially, the anxiety would be less, and it can keep intensifying over a long period. As time passes, your anxiety would keep getting stronger, and it simply doesn't pass away like a panic attack.

- Anxieties are usually followed by a long period of worries. It keeps the mind occupied and leads to overthinking and development of deep fear. Panic attacks end fast, and you will feel all the pressure and fear melting away. You'd feel the intense weight being lifted from your head.

Generalized anxiety in this way is much more dangerous and complex than sporadic episodes of panic attacks. It can last for anywhere between a few minutes to your whole lifetime.

However, every fear and anxiety is not bad. Generally, we feel anxious about things we are not comfortable with. When we are anxious, there can be a rapid pounding of heart, increased pulse, sweating, and tension. You get a general feeling of your inability to cope with a certain situation, and hence defensive mechanism gets activated. Most of the time, people choose to avoid things and situations that may cause anxieties. But, that's not possible in the case of panic attacks as they can come without any such trigger or stressor.

Anxiety disorders should never be ignored as they form the basis of several complicated conditions like social anxiety disorder (SAD), obsessive-compulsive disorder (OCD), posttraumatic stress disorder (PTSD), generalized anxiety disorder (GAD), etc.

Chapter 3: Biological and Psychological Causes of Panic Attacks

Biological Causes of Panic Attacks

There is a lot about the brain and its functioning that modern medical science is yet to discover. We know a lot of things, and we are still in the process of finding out a lot more things. The exact physiological causes of panic attacks are also among the few things medical science is trying to find more about.

The science known until now strongly suggests that panic attacks are caused by the faulty alarm system in our brain.

There is an area in the brain known as Locus Ceruleus. This region has a high concentration of adrenaline-like neurons. The impulse conductors of the nerve cells connect this part to:

- The cerebral cortex (the part of the brain determining intelligence, personality, motor function, senses, etc.)
- The limbic system (responsible for our emotions and higher mental function)
- Thalamus (part of the brain managing pain and emotions)
- Hypothalamus (controls the nervous system and hormone signals)

Effectively, any activity in this part of the brain is going to affect your overall functionality.

This locus ceruleus region and the adrenaline-like neurons can stimulate your body to release hormones that can activate a severe 'fight or flight response.' The body needs this hormone when it is in any kind of danger.

When in danger, the body pumps in adrenaline or epinephrine can make you feel very frightened. In a real-life dangerous situation, that the glucose supply to the cells would be stopped, and all the glucose in the bloodstream would be made available to generate maximum thrust for any action. This simply means that when you are in some grave danger, the power and thrust available to get out of that danger goes up considerably.

This of a scenario where you come face to face with a wild animal. The animal is a quadruped, and hence it has a higher speed than you. In a normal situation, there is no chance for you to outrun that animal. However, due to a very high adrenaline rush in your blood and the resulting fight or flight response, you'll be able to run much faster than your normal capacity to manage survival. This rush is shortlived. It is not possible to manage that speed in normal circumstances, but our body makes a desperate attempt to survive.

This system is there to amplify the chances of survival in dangerous circumstances. Our ancestors had to survive in the wild with no claws, horns, or brute force, whereas the animals were faster, more powerful, and had the accessories like claws, big teeth, and horns. That could make survival difficult, and hence this system was very helpful.

The alarm bells in the locus ceruleus region activate the adrenaline-like neurons, which cause a noradrenergic overload. This is a helpful process in threatening situations. However, in the case of a panic attack, this process gets activated without any stressor or danger trigger. Not only this alarm system gets activated falsely, but it is also very severe in response sending the victim in a state of panic.

Available knowledge and data suggest that this alarm system in our brains is prone to malfunction. Like any alarm system, one or two episodes can occur and then never happen again. This is a reason some people may experience panic attacks once or twice in their lives, never to experience them ever again. Even if you get a panic attack, there is nothing to worry about as just the alarm system has gone off, and otherwise, there is no threat to the body in general. This is a reason panic attacks require no hospitalization or medical care. As there is little understanding of the system, all the causes of the malfunction are not clear, but data shows that hereditary predisposition can make a person prone to such attacks.

There is a high probability that you might have heard the term serotonin. It is commonly used in connection with the things that bring a calming effect to the mind. Instantly after your body has had passed through a severe crisis, you'd notice a feeling of complete relaxation. This feeling of complete relaxation, calm, and peace is brought upon by the effect of serotonin. It is a neuromodulator that helps in modulating anxiety. Gamma-aminobutyric Acid (GABA) is also a neuromodulator chemical. Through several studies, scientists have concluded that when there is a chemical imbalance in the brain, causing low levels of GABA and serotonin, it can lead to panic attacks.

Most theories suggest that the physiological cause of a panic attack somewhere lies in the chemical imbalance in the brain and the faulty alarm system that evokes a crisis response. However, the good thing in these studies is that they suggest this fact with clarity that although the alarm system might be faulty, there is no problem with the basic functioning of the mind and the body.

This means that panic attacks are not a danger for the body. Hence, you don't need to rush to the emergency room every time you have a panic attack or something similar to that. If you could just relax and stay calm, the surge of emotions being experienced by you would pass without an incident.

However, this is easier said than done. The kind of crisis a panic victim feels is only known to that victim. The fear is debilitating. It reduces the victim to nothing. It tears down the personality of the victim. The victims may also face social humiliation due to their sudden reactions. There is no way a panic attack victim can choose the place and time of a panic attack, and that is a reason most victims develop a fear of being in public.

Psychological Causes of Panic Attacks

Panic attacks are strong fear signals being generated in your brain, and your thinking can have a major role to play in that. The kind of temperament you have, the kind of people you socialize with, the kind of job you do, the state of your financial security, etc. are some of the things that can also have a major role in a panic attack.

If any of these things are leading to any kind of insecurity, you can be at risk of a panic attack. You must remember that any kind of major stress in life can lead to a panic attack, and hence leading a balanced life is important.

If you are a person who is sensitive to negative emotions or who cannot handle stressful events, you must work on this aspect of life along with someone who is encouraging and supporting. Fear of things that are very stressful for you can also lead to panic attacks.

Major life events like the demise of a loved one, childhood experience of physical or sexual abuse, or any other such traumatic event recently can also lead to panic attacks.

Abuse of drugs and alcohol can also lead to panic abuse.

Chapter 4: Who Is At a Greater Risk of Panic Attacks?

Anyone can have panic attacks. This is a problem that can strike anyone. Even the marines, who are fitter than the fittest, can suffer from panic attacks. Therefore, if you are fortunate enough to not have experienced any, all you can do is remain cautious. You must remember that even if a panic attack comes, it is a treatable condition.

However, if you fall under any of these categories, you should remain more cautious:

- **Women:** Unfortunately, women have twice the risk of having a panic attack as compared to men. If you are a woman with claustrophobia or any other anxiety disorder, then also your risk of having a panic attack is very high. You'll need to be extra cautious about the things that can cause severe stress.

- **People between 20-29 Age Group:** Although panic attacks can come in any age group, people in the age group of 20-29 years are more likely to experience panic attacks. However, that doesn't mean that people in the younger or older age groups are immune. It can strike at any age.

- **People with a Family History:** As we have already discussed it, if you have someone in your close family with a history of panic attacks or other mental conditions, your risk of having panic attacks can go up.

- **Stressful Life-events:** If you've been through some very stressful life events such as job loss, failure in any big competition, rejection in something crucial, marriage or divorce, or history of abuse, then also the risk of a panic attack will increase.

- **Anxious or Overthinking Attitude:** Some people have anxiety in their attitude. They are never able to feel safe. They always have a lingering fear that something might go wrong. This feeling is even more overpowering when they are sitting at some very pleasant and secure place. It is their mind at play, all the time. Such people are naturally predisposed to panic attacks.

- **Mental Health Illnesses:** If a person has been struggling with generalized anxiety disorder or depression, then the risk of panic attacks will increase.

- **History of Substance Abuse:** Any person with a history of substance abuse will be at a higher risk of panic attacks. Alcohol disorders will also increase the risk many times over.

Chapter 5: Tips to Cope With Panic Attacks When They Strike

You must accept the fact that panic attacks can come. The biggest problem with panic attack victims is that they can't come to terms with the fact that they have panic attacks.

You must realize that you've had a panic attack, and it's okay to have one. You are not the first one and for sure not the last one to have one. Therefore, the best thing to do is to be calm as it is just a phase, and it'd pass away.

Many a time, when someone has a panic attack, the people standing around ask the victim to breathe deeply or be calm and that never really works. It doesn't mean that deep breathing or staying calm are not effective techniques. The victim is simply not in a condition to hear or understand these things. The power to comprehend things said by others during a panic attack goes down. But, if you train your mind and understand the power of deep breathing and other relaxation techniques, you can effectively avoid panic attacks or minimize their severity.

We'll deal with two things in this chapter:

1. Ways to Prevent Panic Attacks
2. Ways to Cope with Panic Attacks

- **Practice Breathing Exercises:** This is probably one of the most important advice you'll ever hear in panic attack prevention. When having a panic attack, the biggest problem faced is breathlessness. The brain starts getting devoid of oxygen. If you practice deep breathing exercises, you'll be able to prevent panic attacks to a great extent. Breathing exercises are very easy and won't take longer than a few minutes of your time daily. You can practice yoga asanas as they are especially very helpful in preventing panic attacks.

- **Light Exercises**: Exercise has a very positive impact on the brain. When you exercise, the body releases hormones called endorphins that help you in relaxing and also induce a happy mood. Regular exercise can promote a sense of positivity in you and help in preventing panic attacks. However, you must remember that this usually helps when you do light exercises. When you are doing strength training and other accelerated stuff, you must be careful when you are hyperventilating as it can trigger a panic attack. In such a circumstance, your priority must remain to catch your breath first.

- **Manage Blood Sugar Levels:** Keeping your blood sugar levels managed is also a way to prevent panic attacks.

- **Avoid Stimulants like Caffeine, Nicotine, and Alcohol:** Most people know that drug abuse can lead to panic abuse, but a large number of people find it hard to believe that excessive amounts of caffeine, nicotine, and alcohol can also trigger panic attacks. You must try to avoid these.

- **Cognitive Behavioral Therapy (CBT):** This therapy can help you identify and change negative thought patterns leading to panic attacks.

Ways to Cope With Panic Attacks

- **Accept and Recognize:** Panic attacks are short, and they are harmless. You must realize the fact that the episodes you experience don't last long. No matter how bad you might feel at that moment, panic attacks pass, and you are safe again. Therefore, there is no need to fear panic attacks or to stay in denial. If you are having a panic attack, you must recognize it. Once you learn to recognize and accept the fact that you are having a panic attack, it'd be easier to understand that they will pass safely.

- **Deep Breathing:** Breathing deeply while you are having a panic attack is always helpful. Shortness of breath or breathing difficulties are common symptoms of panic attacks, and hence deep breathing will not only help in getting over the panic attacks, but it might even prevent a full-blown panic attack even from happening.

- **Inhale Lavender:** Lavender is a stimulant that can help you feel relaxed. If you get panic attacks frequently, you can keep lavender with you and smell a bit of it when having an attack, and it can help you feel relaxed faster.

- **Medication:** Some medications can help you in coping with panic attacks. If you are having panic attacks frequently, you must consult a doctor and take medication for it.

- **Avoid External Stimuli:** Many a time, loud noise in the background, bright lights, or any other kind of stimuli can also accelerate a panic attack. If you feel a panic attack coming, try to find a peaceful place as it can help you focus inwards, and you'll be able to cope with the panic attack better.

- **Try Meditation Techniques:** Meditation is a great way to train your mind to remain peaceful and calm. It is an effective technique to make your mind avoid fearful thoughts or to divert attention from them. If you can practice meditation for a few minutes daily, you'll be able to overcome the problem of panic attacks to a great extent. There are several meditation forms and techniques that you can try. Some of the effective ones are given below:

  o **Mindfulness Meditation:** Most of our panic attacks are either fuelled by our memories of the past or the fears of the future. We are seldom scared of the present as we rarely live in the present. This meditation technique can help you train your mind to live in the present or live mindfully. It can become an effective tool to cope with panic attacks.

  o **Diversion of Mind:** During panic attacks, the mind gets focused on a negative thought. If you can focus your attention on a physical point in front of you and meditate only on that point bringing your complete awareness on it, you will be able to prevent or get over the panic attack faster as your mind will get diverted.

  o **Muscle Relaxing:** Stiffening of muscles and sensation of pain can also act as a trigger for a panic attack. Practicing progressive-muscle relaxation meditation can help you in relaxing the whole body, and it also takes away the mind from fearful thoughts.

o **Picture a Happy Place:** Guided meditation using imagery of a happy place that you can imagine will also help you in coping better from panic attacks. When your mind is thinking about a happy place, it is very relaxed and calm.

o **Use Positive Affirmation:** You can use positive affirmations during a panic attack to reassure yourself that the panic attack will pass shortly without any incident. Positive affirmations like, 'this is a phase, it'll pass,' or 'you are doing fine, there is nothing to worry' can help you in dealing with the panic attacks better.

Chapter 6: The 8-week Plan to Deal With Panic Attacks

Fighting your fears can be a life-long journey. The fears are not physical; they reside in our minds. The more we think about them, the more intense they get. This chapter would help you understand the ways to tackle the things that have been scaring you for all these years.

The plan has been divided into 8 weeks. 1 week for each plan. During that week, you'll have to work only on that specific issue. You may not be addressing the whole problem, but it'll help you in dealing with the issue in the end.

You must understand that the psychology of fear can be ingrained deep inside your mind, and hence it may take you much longer than 8 weeks too. However, no matter how long it takes, if you follow these 8 steps, you'll be able to get the fear of panic attacks due to specific stressors out of your mind.

Week 1

Identify the Triggers, Fears, and Problematic Behavior

When dealing with any kind of problem, it is very important to understand that problem clearly. The biggest problem with panic attacks lies in the fact that you do not know the things causing them. However, that doesn't mean that you are completely oblivious to your fears. Your panic attack is just a sum-total of your fears. If you can identify and address your fears correctly, you'll be able to get rid of them.

Our fears are not random. They originate from various sections of our lives. We may have a fear of things related to work, education, social interaction, or any specific part of these. Once you identify those fears or triggers, dealing with them would be considerably easy. During the first week, you need to analyze every area in your life and note down the things that may be causing stress, fear, or panic. You should be as detailed as possible in this.

Main Areas of Concern:

> **Work-Related:** Most people feel stressed at work. Although that may not cause a panic attack in every individual, there can be some people who might feel highly stressed at their workplace. You should think of all the things at the workplace that make you feel stressed. Try to be very specific. Like if you feel a sense of panic while being called to give a presentation, you must note it down.

> **Social Interaction:** This is another area where many people feel highly insecure. Some people have anxieties about social interaction, and it can cause a panic attack. You must evaluate if social interactions invoke such a reaction in you. Try to be very specific and focused here. Think of the things that might make you feel nervous. Like if being called to sign in a function makes you feel anxious. Most people will feel nervous in that situation, but do you feel a fight or flight response kicking in?

> **Health and Well-being:** People can get anxious thinking about their health or the health of a family member. Think if you have any fear related to that.

Relationship: Think of your fears related to your existing or past relationships and if they are making you feel anxious.

Other Factors: Think of any other fear that might be lingering deep inside you. There can be many other kinds of fears in mind. Some people are afraid of snakes and scorpions; others are scared of allergies; some are scared of heights. Think of the issue that keeps lingering in your mind.

PinPoint the Issue: You must single out the issue. When you have the problem in view, it is always easy to deal with it. Do not try to limit your entry to any specific thing. List all your fears. Try to know everything that has the potential to make you feel anxious or bring a panic attack.

Week 2

Identify Your Negative Thought Patterns

Once you have the list of things that make you fearful, you can move ahead to deal with the thoughts that lead to such fears. The fears do not come from outside. They are an exaggeration of the thoughts we have about them. Some people may faint when asked to give a speech in front of a gathering while others feel themselves at ease doing so. The task was the same for both, but their minds were working in different ways. The fearful mind started thinking about the consequences of giving that speech like being ridiculed, laughed at, talked about behind the back, saying something unreasonable, etc. The fearless mind saw an opportunity to gain popularity and express views. The situation was the same, but different minds made different assumptions and conclusions. You need to keep in mind that the assumptions made by both could have been wrong. The fearless speakers may have got booed; it happens all the time. However, the fearful speakers would have never reached the podium of completed the speech because the presumptions were incorrect, to begin with.

Our fears are caused by our thoughts, and hence it is important to identify negative thought patterns in the mind to deal with those fears.

Negative thought patterns can be classified in the following broader terms:

Unhelpful Thoughts: These are the thoughts that lead to doubts as you start thinking anything. If you are thinking of undertaking a journey, they'll lead you to think about accidents or bad things that may happen on the journey. If you are thinking of applying for a job, these thoughts will make you think about getting rejected and make you experience that feeling. You must identify if you have unhelpful thoughts very often.

What if Thoughts: These are the thoughts that try to analyze every situation. It may seem logical to think of all the sides of the coin, but it isn't as simple as that. These thoughts will lead you to emphasize on the negative outcomes.

Critical Thoughts: These are the thoughts that make you look at the negative side of everything. You become critical of your abilities, and this can start making you feel insecure, leading to panic attacks.

Victimizing Thoughts: These are the thoughts that make you feel like a victim in every situation. The victim mentality can be very dangerous as it kills all kinds of initiative. It makes you feel exploited and vulnerable, and it can lead to panic attacks. You must identify if you have victimizing thoughts.

Know the Way You Think: To solve any problem, you must know the problem first. Your thoughts are the fuel that leads to the rocket of fear that takes you on panic trips. If you want to avoid panic attacks, it is pertinent that you identify your thought pattern. You must know the way your brain thinks, and then only you will be able to make a strategy to break that thought pattern.

Week 3 and 4

Dissociate From the Negative Thought Patterns

Once the task of identifying negative thought patterns has been completed, you need to devise strategies to change those thought patterns. This may take even longer than two weeks.

Thought patterns develop over a very long period. You may have been practicing the same thought pattern since your childhood. Most thought patterns are picked from the surrounding. This solid conditioning makes the breaking of thought patterns a tough and time-consuming task as you'd need a lot of practice.

However, the only way to do this is to practice it over and over again to make this thought pattern a habit.

Practice Labeling Your Thoughts: This is the first thing that you must do. You learn to label the thought. When you have a negative thought in your mind, learn to label it as 'just a thought.' Our mind is conditioned to consider such thoughts as facts since once it is considered a fact, it is easy to believe. You'll have to identify every negative thought and label it as just a thought, and then it'd be easier to work with it. It wouldn't ring in your brain as the gospel truth.

Make It Funny: If there is any such thought that is making you feel insecure, or which is intimidating you, try to say that out in a funny tone. This simple exercise would help you make light of it. That thought wouldn't remain very fearful or intimidating.

Push Positive Thinking to that Thought: Most negative thoughts become powerful because they never get countered by a positive thought. Try countering the negative thought in your mind with a positive idea.

Evaluate that Thought: You must grade every thought as helpful or unhelpful and discard unhelpful ideas. Once you start grading your thoughts, it'd be easier for you to distance yourself from negative thoughts. They wouldn't have command over your mind.

Find time in the future to ponder over it: If any specific thought is still lingering in your mind, find a time in the future to think it over and get it out of the way. Breaking negative thought patterns should be your focus. If there is any thought that's causing trouble in your mind, either counter it positively or get it out of the mind for the time being.

Week 5

Facing the Fears Head-on

Fear is our biggest enemy. Once you have broken the negative thought pattern, your mind will be able to think about things in a much better way. Yet, it may not be ready to shun all fears. If you are faced with situations that filled you with a sense of anxiety previously, they'll have the same impact again. The correct way to face fears is to experience and overcome them. However, this can't be done without preparation.

> **Facing Fears in a Safe Environment:** The best way to move in this direction is to face your fears in a safe environment. If you feel that you have an intense fear of public speaking, begin by speaking only in front of a small group of your friends. When you see that you have a familiar group of faces that is even encouraging you, it'll be easier to give your first speech. Give a few speeches like than and then begin expanding the circle. Include a few people who are friends of friends and then strangers. When you move in a step-by-step manner in a safe environment conquering any fear becomes possible. The key is not to expose yourself to the fearful situation all at once but to do that gradually.

Week 6

Practice Relaxation

Completely relaxing the mind is the key to overcoming panic attacks, but this is just not a psychological process as there is biology involved too. As we have discussed, panic attacks can have some severe symptoms like shortness of breath, nausea, chest pain, etc. All these symptoms emerge because your body has a quick and severe response to a stressor. You must learn to keep the body relaxed to manage panic attacks successfully.

These relaxation techniques can help you in dealing with panic attacks is an amazing way. Not only will you feel more relaxed, but even the recovery from a panic attack would be very much easier.

Practice Relaxation Meditation: Relaxation meditation is the best when it comes to panic relief or relieving stress. It is easy and simple. You can practice it sitting or lying down as you feel comfortable. Just close your eyes and keep your awareness focused on a point. Keep breathing deeply and just push any thought that comes to mind. Your awareness should just focus on the point you are looking at with your eyes closed. Make everything else less important than this. This simple meditation will help you achieve a state of thoughtlessness.

Deep Breathing: This is one of the most important exercises in dealing with panic attacks or any other kind of anxiety. It is very simple and highly effective. You can follow it anywhere anytime. Whenever you feel a panic attack coming, you can start focusing on your breath and begin deep breathing. You'll see that a majority of times, you'll just not have a panic attack. Deep breathing is as simple as its name. Keep taking deep breaths in and then release your breath very slowly. You should also practice it at least once a day.

Progressive Muscle Relaxation: Stiffness of muscles is another cause of panic attacks. The pain and stiffness in the body keep getting ignored and emerges as a negative impulse. An easy way to get rid of that is to follow progressive muscle relaxation techniques. In this meditation technique, you scan your whole body through your awareness and release the pressure and anxiety built up in those areas.

It gives you effective control of your body and also fills you up with a realization that there is no stress or anxiety inside you.

Meditation Using Guided Imagery: This is the best way to manage panic attacks. You can have a recorded guided meditation session using positive imagery liked by you. You'll be free to choose a location or situation of your choice. You can record it yourself or get a pre-recorded one. Whenever you fear a panic attack, you can switch on that guided meditation session, and the recollection of that happy place can help you avoid the negative thoughts that may lead to a panic attack.

Week 7

Practice Mindfulness

This week, you must practice mindfulness. Most people confuse meditation and mindfulness as being interchangeable terms, but they are not. Meditation is the art of looking inside. You don't run away from thoughts, you look inside the thoughts and try to understand them objectively. Mindfulness, on the other hand, is the practice of doing things mindfully. You stop running in an automated mode and start putting your consciousness behind every action you take.

For instance, when you eat, you pay attention to all the aspects of the food. You feel the taste, the aroma, the flavors, and the texture of the food. You pay attention to the process of eating. You chew the food properly and feel it while you chew. This process not only improves your understanding of every process, but it also helps in eliminating any kind of fear present in your mind regarding them.

Some Parts of Mindfulness Practice are:

Meditation: Be meditative in everything you do. Stop doing things in an automated mode. Take cognizance of every action you take.

Be Observant: Observe things more carefully and closely. Don't allow things to pass in front of you like that. Be observant of the things around you.

Stop Before Reacting: Before you react to anything, stop for a moment and think about that thing, the reaction it requires, and the kind of reaction you were going to give.

Learn to Shift Awareness: Learn the art of shifting your awareness on the object of your choice. For instance, if you are having fearful things about your flight, you should be able to fix your awareness at the swiftly moving second hand of your clock or any other such thing.

Week 8

Getting the Experience

This is the week to experience and practice all that you have learned in the past two months. The process may take a bit longer than two months in your case, but there is no need to worry as this is not to scale.

Just go out in the world and face your fear head-on.

However, you must observe the things you have been able to incorporate easily and the things that still need some work.

PART II

Chapter 1: Anxiety, The Monster Within

"I know what it's like to be afraid of your own mind."

- Dr. Reid from Criminal Minds

- Obsessing over small worries that constantly distract you
- Whirling from action to action to try to quiet your minds' nagging
- Attempting to drown out anxious thoughts in any way possible, solemnly wishing they would just disappear

If you are here with us today, you are likely living through all the above and more, trying strategy after strategy to eliminate these causes of stress. Or, perhaps you are seeking help for a loved one that has anxiety that is weighing them down. Or, maybe you are simply here to feed your curiosity of what anxiety is and how it plagues the mind. No matter, I work with anxiety every day and have spent the majority of my existence on Earth immersed in it.

My grandfather was such a worrier that he physically shook, *constantly*. His body would tremble from the overwhelming magnitude of worry that lurked within him. He was a burly southern man who favored anything outdoors and fishing. His long, curly locks framed his rounded face with an always generous smile. When he was at his warmest, he was a magnet to others. However, his most natural state was when he was in worry mode.

What did he worry about? Anything and everything. He was worried about all the typical things that grandparents do; along with I'm sure many countless unspoken things.

"Do you have enough to eat?"

"Do you need the salt or pepper?"

"Are you comfortable? Too hot? Too cold?"

Even though he was a burly man, his voice was soft, so anyone listening had to lean in. I think he like the intimacy it afforded. Whenever we were all at ease, he was at ease.

Us grandkids always ran with the joke, *"Grampy, can we pass you the salt and pepper?"* His anxiousness would disappear with a smile and flush of embarrassment. We did this to show our appreciation, to relieve the tension and let him know he was never a burden and that we loved our big burly gramps for who he was.

Our gramps was a people-person, always curious and invested in others. I have very clear memories of coming home and hearing his low but small voice in the answering machine, *"Hello, it is just me again. Just checking in to see how you are coming along…"*

He needed that regular assurance that everything was, in fact, alright and always preferred to hear it firsthand. And if he could do things for someone, that was even better.

As Gramps aged, his anxiety escalated and he became less able to use it in a constructive manner. There were less and fewer ways for him to release his anxious feelings, to the point he became crippled with worried on a daily basis. When I search into where my own anxiety stemmed from, a picture of Grampy always pops into my mind. When I studied anxiety in graduate school, his shaking body was a perfect analogy. The more time I spent exposed to the study of anxiety in the human body, I began to understand my grandfather better than he likely understood himself most days. I also realized how persuasive anxiety was throughout our family's history. It was what set the foundation for me to deeply understand how much anxiety affected emotions and behaviors.

Thankfully, no one else in my family shook as much as my grandfather did from anxiety; however, looking back, anxiety was the hub of all the spectrum of extremes my family endured. My mother was motivated by her anxiety, while my father was like a balloon, letting stress and anxious feelings build up until he popped with rage.

While no one in my immediate family was ever diagnosed with an anxiety disorder, I can still imagine that just like so many others, they would have felt the same shameful stigma that comes along with all mental health problems, thinking that something is wrong with them. They were simply noticing things in their lives and felt deeply about them; they just didn't have the tools and knowledge to cope with the overload of information.

Through my years as a psychologist, I have gained a different perspective on anxiety and how it alters thoughts and feelings. I have come to see anxiety as a resource and seek to embrace its value in our everyday lives.

Anxiety derives from the feeling of realizing that something we genuinely care about may be at risk, as well as the arrival of resources that we need in order to protect it. Anxiety prompts us to look closer and pay better attention to messages we receive and helps us to gain the motivation we need to take control of situations. The key to getting back a life driven by anxiety and fear is to take control. This is where I have used my knowledge to help others, in ultimately steering them in a different direction of gaining back their willpower.

How Anxiety Overshadows Everyday Lives

Living in denial, second-guessing your every move, thinking ill thoughts about your future, living in fear of the unknown; all these things can overshadow a person's life and lead to constant anxiety.

If you or a loved one is plagued by anxiety, you have probably endured panic attacks and constant negative nagging in your head on a regular basis or have a phobia of some kind feel ashamed of their "sickness."

Anxiety has the power to make everyday folks feel insane, even though they truly aren't. Just like with all people, some days are better than others, but those who experience symptoms caused by these mental ailments typically have a higher count of bad than good days.

They often feel that they are always under a dark cloud that pours rain, but that rain is not made up of just water. Those drops from the sky above their head are created from startling visions, disturbing logic, feelings of worthlessness and/or hopelessness and looks that they receive from both loved ones and strangers when they truly believe they are in a type of personal crisis or feel as if they are about to be pushed over the edge. This is just a small portion of what it is like to live with anxiety.

What is Anxiety?

Anxiety, in its simplest form, is a bodily reaction to unfamiliar or dangerous environments and scenarios. Everyone has the tendency to get anxious from time to time and feel distressed or uneasy. This happens perhaps before a big game, performing in front of an audience or right before a huge job interview. Feeling anxious is a natural response that our bodies can feel during moments like these. Anxiety gives us the boost we need to be consciously aware and alert to prepare us for certain situations.

Our body's "fight-or-flight" response is under this umbrella of reactions. But imagine feeling like this *all* the time, even during the calmest of moments?

Picture a life where you have issues concentrating on everyday tasks, where you may be frightened to leave the safety of your home when you cannot fall or stay asleep because your mind is in a constant whirlwind of thought? Living with an anxiety disorder is debilitating. That is putting it lightly in some cases.

Causes of Anxiety

Every one of us is unique, which means even common disorders, like anxiety and depression, resonate within each of us differently, as well as why we are living with anxiety, to begin with. There are several key factors that cause anxiety disorders to grow in the mind:

- Chemistry of the brain
- Environmental factors
- Genetics
- How we grew up
- Life events

The factors listed above are the basics that lay the groundwork to potentially be a victim of anxiety, but those below mixed with any of those above could set one up to be someone that is at a higher risk than others in the development of an anxiety disorder:

- Alcohol, prescription medication or drug abuse
- Chemical imbalances in the body and/or brain
- History of anxiety that runs in family bloodlines
- Occurrence of other mental health issues
- Physical, emotional or mental trauma
- Side effects one has on particular medications
- Stress that lasts an extended amount of time

The feelings and thoughts that anxiety promotes within a sufferer create a bubble that creates lonely thoughts and feelings, which is why it is no surprise that anxiety disorders are the most common of mental illnesses with the U.S, with **over 40 million American adults** living with one of these disorders as we speak.

If it is any consolation, you are by no means alone when it comes to feeling the way you do. There is still a lot of research being put into finding out why anxiety plagues so many individuals, its specific causes and why it resonates within individuals in such vast ways.

Signs & Symptoms of Anxiety Disorders

All of us will experience anxiety in our lives; it is a normal response to stressful life events. But as you have learned so far or experienced for yourself, these symptoms can become much larger than the events of stress them and can interfere heavily with a happy, healthy way of life.

Below are the most common symptoms of anxiety:

- **Worrying** that is disproportionate to the events that trigger it and is intrusive, making it challenging to concentrate on everyday tasks.
- **Agitation** that causes fast heartrates, sweaty hands, dry mouth, etc.
- **Restlessness** or feeling on edge with a constant uncomfortable urge to move that won't go away.
- Becoming **easily fatigued**, either in general or after a panic attack.
- **Difficulty focusing** on everyday tasks.
- **Issues retaining short-term memory** which results in a lack of performance in multiple areas of life.
- Becoming **easily irritable** in the day to day life.
- Constantly having **tense muscles** that may even heighten anxious feelings.
- **Issues falling and staying asleep** due to continued disturbances in the sleep cycle.
- **Panic attacks** that produce overwhelming sensations of fear.
- **Avoidance of social situations** due to a fear of being judged, humiliated, or embarrassed.

- **Extreme fears** about very specific situations or objects that are severe enough to interfere with normal functioning.

Understanding Social Anxiety

Imagine at random times, feeling so uncomfortable in particular situations to the point of not being able to process what is happening around you or difficulty breathing. Welcome to the life of those that deal with social anxiety. Social anxiety is classified by a major discomfort with social interactions as well as a fear of judgment. There are more than 15 million Americans that deal with this in their everyday lives that struggle with the awkwardness of social settings.

Symptoms of Social Anxiety

The main symptoms of this form of anxiety are feeling intensely anxious when in social situations or avoiding them altogether. Many sufferers have a constant feeling that 'something just isn't right', but are never able to pinpoint it.

As you can imagine, these people have a twisted way of thinking that includes false beliefs of situations and negative opinions from others. Many people fear the interaction days or weeks before the event, which means that social anxiety can manifest in other physical symptoms, such as:

- Sweating
- Shaking
- Diarrhea
- Upset stomach
- Muscle tension
- Blushing
- Confusion

- Pounding of heart
- Panic attacks

The key aspect of social anxiety to remember is that even though these folks have a fear of speaking or interacting with others, it doesn't mean they have nothing to say.

Below are things that those who suffer from social anxiety would say to others to help them understand how they feel:

"I do not want this and I cannot help it. It is not just a bit of nervousness that comes and goes. It is constant stress and living in a world that you start to not recognize."

"In my ability to speak right, I lack confidence. There are many times I want to say something, but hold back because I am afraid of how dumb it may sound or that I will be misunderstood. I am afraid of speaking in groups, phone calls, and approaching people the most.

"I am terrified of people's reactions when I do scrounge up the courage to finally speak."

"My anxiety socially is not a constant. There are certain situations that cause me more anxiety than others. It is a fluid disease."

"Many times, people don't realize that those with this anxiety disorder are suffering because of the lack of physical symptoms. Just because you cannot tell there is something wrong, doesn't mean there isn't."

"I cannot help how ridiculous it may seem."

"It hurts to know that people take my anxiety personally instead of just helping me out."

"I wish I had a social life, but my anxiety won't let me; I am not anti-social."

"It may look like I am zoning out from time to time, but I am actually practicing positive self-talk and breathing techniques to stay calm and ward off a panic attack."

"I am not trying to be standoffish, rude, or snobby, even though it may seem that way when I refuse hugs or don't wish to speak. I simply get overwhelmed and overstimulated easily. All I ask for is respect."

"I want people to break the ice and speak to me first. I am genuinely a nice person, I just

have a fear I am unable to control."

"I wish more people understood that when I say I cannot come, it is because the situation I was invited to feels 'impossible', not because I don't feel like it."

"When I leave early, I am not being disrespectful. I just need to fight off a meltdown with some alone time."

"Social anxiety is not 'shyness'; that is like comparing a stab wound to a paper cut."

No one experiences social anxiety in the same way. Each day is like living a life of constant fear; worrying about the disapproval of others, rejection, not fitting in, etc. They are bound to be anxious to enter or begin a conversation.

Chapter 2: Acknowledging Your Anxiety

While the numbers of those that suffer from anxiety in the United States alone exceed 40 million, you may feel alone in your symptoms as well as what triggers them. Things that set off those anxious thoughts and feelings are a bit different for everyone who experiences anxiety. It is important to take time to focus on yourself and learn what things provide you with peace or create tension in your life.

Common Anxiety Triggers

- The hustle and bustle of everyday life. Life is always busy and there never seems to be time to slow down.
- The inevitable fact that we are only growing older.
- Driving, especially on freeways with many cars or across bridges.
- Not living up to the expectations that we set for ourselves.
- The sense of uncertainty. When we are not on control of situations we tend to freak out a bit. This comes from a lack of communication and anxiety making conclusions for us.
- Ambulance, fire or police sirens.
- Stresses at work – Not performing well enough, not having enough time during the course of the workday to get things done, etc.
- Simply thinking about what triggers your anxiety can be a cause for anxiousness in itself.
- Being too hot is often times directly associated with being claustrophobic.
- The inevitable part of life known as death. This especially goes for individuals who have experienced much loss in their lives.
- Being alone.

- The possibility of finding out that people do not like you as much as you think they do.
- Being judged or verbally attacked.
- Large crowds.
- The inability to predict the future. Those with anxiety often dislike surprises.
- Trying new things.
- Being far away from home or other places familiar to you.
- When many people speak to or at you all at once.
- The struggles that your children may face at school.
- Money! This is a big one. Whether it is saving for a big event such as a wedding or purchasing a home or car, the process of paying monthly bills while still trying to save money for other things.

Getting to the Root Causes of Your Anxiety

What many of us do not realize is that many causes that trigger our anxieties to flare up are actually self-produced. While you can blame your situation, family, friends, etc. for you distress, you are the one who perceives life as it goes on around you. The way you view it, analyze and take it all is all dependent on you. The root reasons behind the curtains of 'Play Anxiety' are usually caused by one of the following reasons.

Negative Self-Talk

It is said by research conducted by behavioral specialists that upwards of 77% of all the things we think to ourselves is quite counterproductive and negative. What we don't realize is that we are being our own worst critic and a detriment to ourselves. Learn to become consciously aware of the way you speak to yourself.

Write down any sort of negative thoughts for a day and then each day forward practice transforming those negative words or thoughts into a happy, loving one towards yourself. While it may feel weird at first, it will become second nature to you once you practice it for a while. Your self-talk is just as important of a daily habit as any other.

Unrealistic Expectations

Sometimes we simply just have too high of expectations that create a high world that we struggle to reach. Expecting those to be perfect and remember all the details about you is just ridiculous. If your expectations fly way above you, you are more than likely missing out on grand opportunities and are unable to truly recognize the good things that are happening that you should be celebrating.

This goes for the expectations you have for yourself as well. Are they actually realistic? If not, how can you go about making them more reasonable and achievable?

The "Should" Thoughts

Do you find your brain thinking that you "should do this" and you "should do that" often? Have you ever just taken a moment to actually find the reasoning behind why you "should"? Telling yourself that you should is equivalent to telling yourself that you are not good enough. It leads to negative self-talk fast and should be avoided. Make a positive list of the things you should do or become. Are they yours or someone else's expectations?

Taking Things Too Personally

Those with anxiety feel like many things that occur are actually their fault when in reality they more than likely had nothing to do with someone's disgruntled behavior or a glare they received. Learn to not take things too personally because you never know what may be happening in the life of other people.

"We are all in the same game, just different levels. Dealing with the same hell, just at different devils." If you think you are the cause of someone's actions, speak up and ask instead of just assuming. This will get rid of a lot of assumptions that go into negatively feeding your anxiety.

Our minds are wired to believe the things that we tell it the most. If we are always engaging in negative self-talk, expect too much of others or ourselves, do things we just merely think we "should" do or worry about those around you, your brain will act negatively as well. It is all about building a positive foundation for your frame of mind for all those thoughts of yours to dwell in. In order to unlock the door to happiness and less stress and/or anxiety, it is time to get thinking in a happy manner!

Pinpointing Your Anxiety

While you can take all the time in the world to read information in regards to relieving anxiety via the internet, books or other media, unless you take action and decide that you truly want to make a change to lower your anxiousness, it will never happen. I am an anxiety sufferer and back just a couple years ago it engulfed my everyday life and drowned me more than a few times.

I finally over time came up with a process that assisted me greatly with determining what triggered my anxious thoughts so that I could get a grip on my life and yield them from continuously taking over my personal life.

- **Stop** – When those feeling of anxiousness begin to hit you, stop and take a moment to make a mental note of what you are doing right at that moment. This is easier said than done, for you might be in the middle of a task, conversation, etc. But it is beneficial to take just a moment to identify when you began to feel anxious.

- **Identify** – Recognizing the onset of anxiety will help you come to the conclusion of what actually causes it for you personally. If you develop the capability to notice triggers and feelings when they start to dwell, you can put a stop to them faster. Many people don't realize they are feeling anxious until their symptoms are outrageously taking over them. Over time, you will be able to catch on more quickly what is threatening your happiness and overall well-being.

- **Write** – As you become an expert of taking moments to make mental notes of why you feel anxious, I find that at the end of the day I write down the events during my day, both the goods one and those that triggered my anxiety. I keep a notepad on my cellular device so that I am quickly able to access it to jot down notes at the moment and then write them down on paper before heading to bed. Be sure to write down as many details as possible – what you are thinking, experiencing and feeling, etc.

- **Analyze** – At the end of the week is when I choose to review what I have written in my anxiety notebook. You can review it at the end of each day, week or month, but I do not recommend waiting any longer than that. I wait at least a couple days to a week so that I can see the pattern that my thoughts made. When you are aware of these patterns you are better able to focus on the causes of anxiety and avoid them.

- **Possibilities** – There are numerous things that you can make the scapegoat when it comes to feeling anxious. If you have adequate knowledge of these ideas, you can review patterns and conquer anxiety. Anxiety in many cases is situational. If you are anxious being in unfamiliar surroundings, expose yourself to these types of circumstances a little time. If your causes are more based on the way you think and view the world, learn to engage in positive self-talk. Once you have a pattern written out, you will be less anxious just by the fact that you have some idea and control over your anxiety situation overall.

Chapter 3: Trauma and Anxiety

The journey of life is exciting, scary, ridiculous, confusing and worth it all at once. But there are times that we all go through some type of emotional distress, whether it be mere sadness, rapid anxiety, addictions to outside influences, obsessions with things or people, compulsions we have a hard time controlling, behaviors that are self-sabotaging, physical injuries, anger, and bleak moods, among the hundreds of other things we go through, think and/or feel.

It is important to learn ways to cope when it comes to hard times, no matter the time frame. Something psychologically downgrading can happen in a matter of mere moments and leave you scarred for the rest of your life. Some people seek out help from other individuals who are professionals at understanding the human mind, but others wish to find help within them. Having the knowledge to help yourself is not an easy feat. It may be easy to read pages upon pages of books and self-help websites that provide information, but it is much harder to put those words into actions.

The world is a much different place now than it was just a decade or two ago. Technology has advanced so rapidly that some of us are overwhelmed with it all, especially the consequences that we receive, whether from our own actions or that of another being who acted upon a current mood. Human beings are not the robots that we seem to want to create so badly these days. We are emotionally driven individuals with a lack of having the knack to help ourselves in times of need and/or trouble.

The worst thing about the constant rise of this distress is the fact that there is no one age group or certain targeted individuals that are more likely to go through it. It is happening clear from late grade school levels all the ways into senior living years. Students have much more stress with perpetual levels of testing and pressure to be better. Employees live their hard-earned careers always fighting to make their way up the ladder with not much reward. Older individuals are continuously having their wages and retirement that they worked their entire lives for whisked away.

It is a dog eat dog world out there with a lot of room to make mistakes that can cause even more friction in our personal lives. With the constant pressure to be better than the next, our society has taught us maybe how to be more proficient in terms of getting things done at school or work, but many of us have forgotten the person that is truly important: OURSELVES. If we do not take care of our emotional health, detrimental things can occur. Below are some signs that you may be experiencing emotional distress. Some of the symptoms may surprise you.

Childhood Trauma and Sensitivity to Anxiety

Trauma during childhood can impact our entire lives. According to the Journal of Affective Disorders, children who experience traumatic situations are much more likely to have anxiety and depressions and fall victim to alcohol and drug abuse. The same study found that females are more susceptible than males to develop anxiety, even with the same rates of trauma.

If left untreated, trauma during childhood can have effects that last throughout someone's entire life. They are likely to developmental disorders that branch out to much more than just anxiety as well.

Common Anxiety Disorders Caused by Trauma

Common anxiety disorders that are caused by traumatic events are:

- Panic disorder
- Obsessive Compulsive Disorder (OCD)
- Post-Traumatic Stress Disorder (PTSD)
- Body Dysmorphic Disorder

- Agoraphobia
- Social Phobia(s)

As you can imagine, trauma anytime throughout your life can play a major part in the development of anxiety and other mental disorders in your lifetime.

Chapter 4: Grabbing your life back from anxiety

Now that you have acknowledged that life could be better and have learned how to interpret why you live a life filled with anxiety, it is time to take your life back, pronto! There is a variety of methods we will discuss in this chapter that can help you gain back the confidence you need to live life to the fullest.

Managing Your Emotions

Emotions are a natural human phenomenon. , and are very present in pressing and painful times. Every day we are driven by some force of emotions:

- We take chances because we get excited about new opportunities
- We cry because we are hurting and make sacrifices for those we love

Those are just a couple examples of emotions; they dictate our actions, intentions, and thoughts with authority to our rational minds. Emotions can become a real problem, however, when we act too fast or we act on wrong types of emotions, which cause us to make rash decisions.

Negative emotions, such as bitterness, envy, or rage, are the ones that tend to spiral out of control the most, especially when triggered. It only takes one slip of our emotions to totally screw up the relationships in our lives.

If you have issues controlling your emotions, here are some steps that you can implement into your everyday life that will help you regain rationality, no matter what challenging situation you are facing:

Don't react right away

You are more likely to make mistakes when you react right away to emotional triggers. When reacting right away to these triggers, you are likely to say and do things that you will later regret.

Before acting on emotions, take a deep breath to stabilize your impulses.

Breathe deeply for just a couple minutes and you will be able to feel your heart rate return to normal. One you become calmer, remind yourself that feeling this way is just temporary.

Find healthy outlets

Once you have managed your emotions, you need to learn how to release that build up in the healthiest way possible; emotions are something that you should never let bottle up. Talk to someone you trust. Hearing their opinion of the matter can help to broaden your thoughts and regain control.

Many people keep a journal to write down how they feel. Others engage in exercise to discharge their emotions. Others meditate in order to return to their tranquil state. Whatever activity suits you, find it and use it when emotions get high.

Look at the bigger picture

All happenings in our, both bad and good, serves a purpose in our lives. Being able to see past the moment strengthens your wisdom. You may not understand certain circumstances right away, but over time, you will see the bigger picture as the pieces of the puzzle fall into order. Even when in an emotionally upsetting time, trust that there is a reason that you will comprehend in time.

Replace your thoughts

Negatively fueled emotions create negative recurring thoughts that create cycles of negative patterns over time. When confronted with these emotions, force them out of your mind and replace them with more positive thoughts. Visualize the ideal ending playing out or think about someone or something that makes you happy.

Forgive your triggers

Triggers could be the ones you love the most; you're best friend(s), your family, yourself, etc. There will be times that you may feel a sudden wave of rage when people do things that annoy you or a self-loathing feeling when you remember back to the past when you could have done thing differently. The key to managing your emotions is to first, forgive. This allows you to detach from your jealousy, fury, and resentment. As you forgive, you will discover that disassociating yourself from these feelings will do you the best.

Every day we are constantly reminded of how strong and prominent our emotions are and the power they have. We are bound to take the wrong action from time to time and feel the wrong things. To avoid acting out, simply take a few steps back and calm your spirit that is heightened from outside forces. You will be grateful for mastering your emotions when it comes to building and strengthening meaningful relationships.

Using the Power of Mini Habits

Just after Christmas in the days ending 2016, I was reflecting on the year. I realized that I had tons of room to improve but always failed at keeping up with my New Year's resolutions. Instead, I decided that in 2017, I would explore other options.

On the 28th of December, I made the choice that I wanted to get back in shape. Previously, I hardly if ever exercised and had a consistent guilt about it. My goal was a 30-minute workout, realistic, right?

I found myself unmotivated, tired, and the guilt made me feel worthless. It wasn't until a few days later that I came across a small blog article about thinking the opposite of the ideas you are stuck on. The clear opposite of my 30-minute workout goal was chilling on the couch, stuffing my face with junk food, but my brain went to the idea of 'size.'

What if, instead of carrying that guilty feeling around all the time, I just performed one push-up? I know, right? How absurd of me to think that a single push-up would do anything to help me towards my goal.

What I found was a magical secret to unlocking my potential…when I found myself struggling with my bigger goals; I gave in and did a push-up. Since I was already down on the floor, I did a few more. Once I performed a few, my muscles felt warmed up and I decided to attempt a pull-up. As you can imagine, I did several more. And soon, I exercised for entire 30-minutes!

What Are Mini Habits?

Mini habits are just like they sound; you choose a habit you want to change and you shrink them down to stupidly small tasks.

For instance, if you want to start writing at least 1,000 words per day:

- Write 50 words per day

- Read two pages of a book per day

Easy, right? I could accomplish this in 10 to 20 minutes or so. You will find that once you start meeting this daily requirement, you will far exceed them faster than you would imagine.

What is *More* Essential than Your *Habits*?

You might be wondering how you can become more comfortable in your skin and be yourself in a cruel world with these so-called mini habits. Well, think about it; what is more important than the things you do each and every day? NOTHING. Habits are responsible for 45% of how we behave, making up the foundation of who we are and how happy we are in life.

The main reason people fail to change anything in their life, even the aspects they know need to change is because they never instill new habits. Why? Simply because in the past, they have tried to do way too much, all at once. If establishing a new habit requires you to have more willpower than you can muster, you are bound to be unsuccessful. If a habit requires less willpower, you are much more likely to succeed!

Benefits of Mini Habits

There are many additional benefits that come with utilizing mini habits in your everyday life. Here are a few:

- Consistent success breeds more success
- No more guilt
- Stronger productivity
- Formation of more positively impactful habits
- Generation of motivation

Chapter 5: Belittle anxiety with personal empowerment

Having a negative attitude towards life keeps us from being happy and impacts those that we interact daily with. Science has more than enough proof to show how being positive impacts your levels of happiness and terms of success. This is why making positivity a habit with the help of small changes can help you to drastically change your overall life and the mindset you have towards the world. The life you are living is a direct reflection of your overall attitude. It can be quite easy, almost too easy, to be cynical at the world and see it as a mess of injustice and tragedy, especially thanks to the media that we all spend many hours a day on.

Negativity is holding you back from really enjoying your life and has a great impact on your environment as well. The energy that people bring to the table, including you, is very contagious. One of the best things you can do in your life that is free of charge and simplistic is to offer your positive attitude. This is especially beneficial in a world that loves and craves negativity.

One of my favorite quotes of all time comes directly from the King of Pop, Michael Jackson: "*If you want to make the world a better place, take a look at yourself and make a change.*"

As humans, we are creatures of habit. In this chapter, we will outline small but significant changes that can be made to form positive habits that can drastically change the overall mindset of your life around.

Smile

When asked who we think about most of the time, the most honest answer would probably have to be ourselves, right? This is natural, so don't feel guilty! It is good to hold ourselves accountable and take responsibility for ourselves.

But I want to challenge you to put yourself aside for at least one moment per day (I recommend striving for more) and make another person smile.

Think about making someone else happy and that warm feeling you get when you receive happiness. We don't realize how intense the impact of making someone smile can have on those around us. Plus, smiling costs nothing and positively works your facial muscles!

Focus on solutions, not problems

Embracing positivity doesn't mean you need to avoid issues, but rather it is learning how to reconstruct the way you criticize. Those that are positive create criticisms with the idea to improve something. If you are just going to point out the issues with people and in situations, then you should learn to place that effort instead into suggesting possible solutions. You will find that pointing out solutions makes everyone feel more positive than pointing out flaws.

Notice the rise, not just the downfall

Many of us are negative just by the simple fact that we dwell too much on the hate and violence that is in our daily media. But what we fail to notice is those that are rising up, showing compassion, and giving love to others. Those are the stories you should engulf yourself in. When you able to find modern-day heroes in everyday life, you naturally feel more hopeful, even in tough times.

Just breathe

Our emotions are connected to the way we breathe. Think about a time that you held your breath when you were in deep concentration or when you are upset or anxious. Our breath is dependent on how we feel, which means it also has the power to change our emotions too!

Fend off other's negativity

I'm sure you have gone to work cheerful and excited to take on the day ahead, but then your co-worker ruins that happy-go-lucky mood of yours with their complaints about every little thing, from the weather to other employees, to their weekend, etc.

It is natural to find yourself agreeing to what others are saying, especially if you like to avoid conflict. But you are initially allowing yourself to drown in their pool of negative emotions. Don't fall into this trap.

Conflict may arise, but I challenge you to not validate the complaints of a friend, family member, or co-worker next time they are going about on a complaint-spree. They are less likely to be negative in the future if they have fewer people to complain to.

Switch the "*I have to*" mindset with "*I get to*"

I am sure you often fail to notice how many times we tell ourselves that we have to go and do something.

- "I have to go to work."
- "I have to go to the store."
- "I have to pay rent."
- "I have to mow the lawn."

You get the picture. But watch what happens when you swap the word have with the word get.

- "I get to go to work."
- "I get to go to the store."
- "I get to pay rent."
- "I get to mow the lawn."

See the change in attitude there? It goes from needing to fulfill those obligations to be grateful that you have those things to do in your life. This means:

- You have a job to go to
- You have enough money to support yourself and your family to provide a healthy meal
- You have a roof over your head
- You have a nice yard

When you make this simple change, you will begin to feel the warmth of happiness snuggle you like the cold blanket of stress falls away.

Describe your life positively

The choice of vocabulary we use has much more power over our lives than we realize. How you discuss your life is essential to harnessing positivity since your mind hears what you spew out loud.

When you describe your life as boring, busy, chaotic, and/or mundane, this is exactly how you will continue to perceive it and it will directly affect both your mental and physical health.

Instead, if you describe your life as involved, lively, familiar, simple, etc., you will begin to see changes in your overall perspective and you will find more joy in the way you choose to mold your entire life.

Master rejection

You will need to learn to become good at being rejected. The fact of the matter is, rejection is a skill. Instead of viewing failed interviews and broken hearts as failures, see them as opportunities for practice to ensure you are ready for what is to come next. Even if you try to avoid it, rejection is inevitable. Don't allow it to harden you from the inside out.

Rethink challenges

Stop picturing your life being scattered with dead-end signs and view all your failings as opportunities to re-direct. There are little to no things in life that we have 100-percent control over. When you let uncontrollable experiences take over your life, you will literally turn into mush.

What you can control is the amount of effort you put into things without an ounce of regret doing them! When you are able to have fun taking on challenges, you are embracing adventure and the unknown, which allows you much more room to grow, learn and win in the future.

Write in a gratitude journal

There are bound to be days where just one situation can derail the entire day, whether it be an interaction that is not so pleasant or something that happens the night before the day ahead, our mind clings to these negative aspects of the day.

I am sure you have read on multiple sites about how keeping a gratitude journal is beneficial. If you are anything like me, I thought this was total rubbish that is until I started doing it. I challenged myself to write down at least five things that I was truly grateful for each and every day. Scientifically, expressing gratitude is linked to happiness and reducing stress.

I challenge you to begin jotting down things you appreciate and are grateful for each day. Even on terrible days, there is something to be blessed about!

Chapter 6: Everyday techniques to fend off anxiety

Despite the toll that anxiety and its symptoms can have on everyday life and fulfillment, in today's world there are many different techniques and methods you can learn to incorporate into your everyday routine that help you to control and possibly even eliminate anxiety from your life. Each section of this chapter will be dedicated to a specific genre of techniques that anyone has the ability to learn!

Visualization and Anxiety

Seeing *is* believing, which is a key secret to how entrepreneurs and well-known people in society stand out and achieve success and fulfill their dreams. *Visualization is the simple use of imagination through mental imagery to help form visions of what we want in our lives and how we can make them a reality.*

There are two main kinds of visualization:

Pragmatic Visualization represents a set of days that helps to gain new ideas and interpret what it says/means to them. It helps those understand structures that lie within a set of data.

Artistic Visualization is similar to pragmatic in that it utilizes visuals to convey information but in a different sense. It is used to show people that data is being monitored carefully and shows particular aspects of data that is connected to one another to depict an entire idea.

So, how does learning about these two kinds of visualization help you in your quest to decrease anxiety? Well, visual techniques help to drastically overcome symptoms of anxiety. When the two types are combined, visualization is powerful in obtaining and staying in a calmer state of mind.

When it comes to anxiety, visualization requires one to picture themselves in a safe, peaceful and/or tranquil environment. Anywhere that makes you happier is where you should be imagining yourself during visualization exercises. It does sound pretty funny at first glance, but trust me when I say there is something about being able to transport your mind to somewhere mentally tranquil. Not only will your mind thank you but your body will too, for it becomes much more relaxed and stress-free when performing these practices. Visualization gives people something to distract themselves from the current world that surrounds them.

Why You Should Be Using Visualization

Beyond visualization itself, you can literally view the best of life from the comfort of your own couch. This chapter will showcase the benefits that come with the dedicated practice of learning and incorporating ways of visualization into your everyday life.

- **Improved quality of relationships** – The positive outcomes of utilizing visualization doesn't just end within yourself. Since you are developing a better mindset that aids in your views and beliefs, those around you will like and appreciate the more confident, positive you!

- **Boosts your mood** – When one practices the methods of visualization, they naturally experience a sort of joy that is quite unexplainable to some. Once you finish one of these sessions successfully, you will more than likely feel boastfully happy, calm and relaxed.

- **Relieves stress** – Practicing the ways of visualization naturally causes one to be able to relax. It has a way of quieting the mind to be able to think happier, more positive thoughts which tone down loads of stress that pile on our shoulders almost on a daily basis.

- **Strengthens the immune system** – Thanks to all that dialing down of stress and things that fuel stress, your body is better able to fight off sickness which makes you physically better, longer. This also helps in aiding anxiety because you are not constantly worrying about getting ill all the time as well.

- **Ability to learn new things quicker** – When the mind is in a calmer state, it is able to pick up and grasp new concepts much easier than when it is bogged down with so many negative thoughts and emotions.

- **Able to cope with the feeling of nervousness** – When you take time out of your day to practice visualization, you are initially settling all those negative feelings that you may have about yourself and what others may think of you as well. This immensely helps individuals who are naturally more nervous combat that feeling, which leaves room to try and experiment with new things and ideas. Imagine yourself in a great looking outfit giving that inevitable speech that is due soon. Then imagine an applauding audience. It is quite the confidence booster!

- **Builds stronger concentration skills** – Visualization makes room for your mind to do other tasks efficiently by spring cleaning negative thoughts, feelings, emotions, and past experiences. This doesn't mean it is responsible for getting rid of them 100%, but it helps one to be able to cope and bring down those bad levels to make room for productivity.

- **Assists in overcoming recurring issues** – When the weight of your entire world is upon your shoulders, it is no wonder that we begin to believe that our lives were just made to be a laughing-stalk to some because of how life's unlucky events have left us feeling. This can lead to long-term problems and beliefs. Visualization combats these two things.

- **Can give you a spark of inspiration** – During your sessions, if your mind always veers to one idea in particular, perhaps it is time to take initiative and proceed with the steps in achieving it! Visualizing doing something can directly inspire you to do as such.

- **Makes one more creative** – Visualization not only takes concentration but also a truckload of creativity as well. If you are going to picture something in detail and add the other four senses to that visual, you have to really want to mold it into reality. We all have creative bones in our bodies. Visualization just brings them out more, honing that skill and letting it shine.

- **No boundaries** – As I have mentioned before, when it comes to visualization, practice makes perfect. Just like with any newly acquired skill, one must learn to hone its practice to be able to tweak it when needed and use it to their utmost advantage. With certain visualization techniques, you can literally picture yourself doing something that would otherwise be usually hard to achieve. With those images in mind, you then have a good idea what you must do to actually and realistically accomplish that image you had in your head during a visualization session. This method knows no bounds!

- **Method of practice and rehearsal** – Believe it or not, visualization can be a way to practice your favorite sport or nail that upcoming work pitch that you have been reciting and memorizing for days. Picturing yourself doing or performing something is just as effective as actually completing the task at hand. Utilizing visualization with real, physical practice can get you to honing that skill or memorizing things much quicker.

- **Picture yourself getting stronger and healthier** – Sounds unbelievable, but if you are sick, seeing yourself get better will have the result of getting healthier, sooner. Visualization reduces stress and relaxes your mind, which also assists in healing your body of sickness or physical injury as well. This allows your body to function at its full capacity. You would be surprised what our bodies could accomplish in a day's work if we treated them more like the temples they are and should always be. It is safe to say we take our physical presence for granted most days. And it tends to show more often than not!

- **Gives us joy** – Many people who practice the ways of visualization tend to picture something that brings them happiness. We almost are never quite in the right place or time in our lives to always have what we want and that is okay! But that doesn't mean we shouldn't get the luxury of seeing it for ourselves, right? Picturing a goal or what we want the most from life can bring us quite a load of temporary happiness if one wants to view it that way. Why temporary? If you can picture it, you can eventually and more than likely make it happen in your future, which is why visualization can be a great motivator.

Aspects of Successful Visualization Practices

There are three aspects to successfully become one with visualization:

- **Practice** – Learning the ways of visualization may actually be more stressful and frustrating for beginners because it is not a practice we are naturally keen to perform. Those that start practicing visualization have a false sense of what the experience is supposed to feel like and have false expectations about the outcome. This inhibits the practice from really taking effect. Visualization is something that has to be practiced daily to work for you long-term. If practiced the right way, it will eventually become second nature to you but only if you really dedicate yourself to learning its ways and practicing it every day until you have it down pat.

- **Utilizes ALL the senses** – Visualization doesn't just use your sense of how a certain peaceful place appears to you in your mind. You have to imagine what your safe space smells, tastes sounds and feels like as well. The more detailed you are in regards to your senses, the better visualization you will have and the more relaxed you can potentially become.

- **Actions** – All human beings experience mental barriers that keep them from being happy and the process of practicing and performing visualization is not excluded from this. Even for visualizing experts, bad thoughts from the course of one's day can inhibit one from getting a clear vision of their safe haven. You have to find a way to release and/or transform those bad thoughts and feelings into something that you can tangibly get rid of.

Forms of Visualization for Anxiety

Visualization is a skill that can be utilized to obtain a better life, especially for those that suffer from an anxiety disorder. Now, we will talk about techniques in the visualization world. Although all of these are not for everyone, try them out and see what works for you.

Meditation

Meditation is a superb form of apathetic visualization that can lead to very powerful results. Visualizing through means of meditation is more of an outgrowth than the main focus. When you begin to incorporate meditation sessions into your everyday routine, you will gradually be opening the door to your inner self, which will then lead you to be able to visualize more clearly and easily.

The more experience you have with meditation, the smoother sessions become and the more you get to see and take away from your visions. It is important not to become frustrated with yourself or discouraged from continuing to practice meditation if you are just starting out.

The whole point of meditation is to empty your brain of thoughts and feelings and to let your mind wander to wherever it wants to go. A vital component of meditation is breathing. Learn to focus on how you take in and let out breaths of air. Let your mind veer off to wherever its little heart desires. Once you begin to practice this technique more often, it will become easier and faster to exhaust your mind of concerns or other worries and let other things come in and explore. It will become second nature for you to sit down, relax and get into a clear state of mind so that you can visualize to your contentment.

Meditation makes way for things that you never thought were actually within you. Once you rid your brainwaves of all that noise from the course of your day, thoughts occur at their own pace.

Altered Memory Visualization

This visualization technique targets past memories and learning how to change them to a more positive standpoint. For those with anxiety about things that stem from their past, this is especially helpful in obtaining a brighter state of mind. This technique is one to utilize if you are one that holds on to past anger and resentment from particular situations that you finally want to rid yourself of.

No one can change the past, but you can teach your brain how it views these past scenarios in your mind. Get into a calmed state and visualize the scenario that you wish had a different outcome. Restore things said that were fueled by anger with comments that are controlled and peaceful. This does take some time and you may have to revisit this scene in your head multiple times to nail the outcome that you wish had resulted from the past situation. It is recommended to not do this day upon day in a row, but rather space out revisiting the scene.

Over time, your brain will begin to only recall what YOU have recreated, making a once painful or uncomfortable situation fade away in memory. Try to imagine little cubicle offices in each major section of your brain. In this instance, I like to picture a little office guy that is in charge of just the bad memories. During these sessions, you are instructing him on how to rewrite particular events that have occurred in the past and once they are rewritten the way you once anticipated them to play out, this office dude can start to shred your memories of these occurrences.

Receptive Visualization

This technique is much like viewing a movie inside your head, but you are the director of the scenes within this movie. Get yourself to a quiet space, lie back, get comfortable and close your eyes. Focus on building the scene in which you want to see acted out in your mind.

Once a clear backdrop and scenery is within your mind, place people, noises, smells and sounds within your scene of this movie. It is best to slowly build your way up to the actual scene until you are comfortable and content with it, then it is time for action! Focus on feeling involved within this scene of your "movie."

Treasure Map

This visualization technique not only uses mental fundamentals but also physical components as well. You will need to have an idea of what you want to visualize before getting to the nitty-gritty of performing this method. Start by using your art skills to draw out some type of physical representation of the components you need to achieve in order to reach your ultimate goal. For example, perhaps you have an upcoming test that you want to get a great grade on. Draw out a building symbolizes a school, a book that you will need to use to study for this test and then a representation of yourself. Try to make your drawing detailed, but do not worry about the maturity of your art abilities too much here. It is not the drawings themselves that are important, but rather what you are imagining WHILE sketching them out.

As you draw out your "map to success", your mind is actually visualizing ways that will get you to where you want to be. Patience is a key with this particular technique, for it does take a bit of time to truly become completely mentally occupied in this exercise. It is crucial to take your notepad and pen to a quiet space and to not be around anything distracting such as a radio, television, people or phones.

How to Design Your Own "Safe Space"

Safe places or spaces are a mind's sanctuary, created for the purpose of retreat if one needs a mental location to be able to visualize or hone their meditative state and reduce stress. Creating one of these is kind of like personalizing a physical space in your home. You want to do anything to truly make it YOURS.

It can be anything from a room inside an imaginary home, a room in your realistic home that you want to visualize differently, the beach, a comforting outdoorsy area, etc. As you meditate or relax and begin to dive deeper into your imagery or visualization session, this is the place you imagine you want to go. It is anywhere that you wish to return to time after time, so put some effort and thought into where you will always find comfort in mentally retreating to.

- **Brainstorm** – The goal is to develop a place that you feel calm, content and happy within, no matter the reason that you retreat to it. If you have difficulty seeking out such a place, start by looking through art, magazines, books, old photographs, etc. Always lean towards ideas that burst with positivity for you.

  - Are you more apt to feel calmer in an outdoor/natural setting or do you feel better within the walls of some type of structure?

  - Are there pieces of writing such as within books, poems of stories that make you feel at ease?

  - Do you feel more comforted by populated areas or tranquil areas?

- **Think of a time where you felt happy and safe** – Memories are the best areas to seek things that bring joy to you. Think back to memories that you were happy, content, playful, peaceful, etc. Write these down in detail. It could be literally anywhere, as long as it brought contentment to you.

  - Where did this memory occur?
  - How old were you?
  - Why did this memory make you happy?
  - Who was with you within this memory?

- **Create various rooms** – Your safe space does not necessarily have to be just 2D, one room vision. It can have various sections, compartments or rooms within it. This allows you to trek to different areas throughout your visualization sessions. This also allows one the ability to be able to compartmentalize issues and deal with them one part at a time.

- *Fill your space with cherished people* – There are many individuals that would rather be alone while in their safe place, while others prefer the company of their favorite people. Imagine who makes you happy and during the course of a visualization session, imagine greeting them and welcoming them into your safe space. This also goes for people in your life that may have passed away that you miss and wish to see. Having conversations with them and asking for advice could make a world of difference!

- *Utilize ALL your senses* – Seeing is believing, but visions of your safe place are a lot more believable and turn in better results if you learn to engage all your senses while within them. Engulf yourself in tastes, sounds smells and how things feel between your fingers and toes and against your skin. It will enhance your visualization experience ten-fold.

- *Write out all the details* – Once you have taken the dedicated time to develop and build your safe place, write down all the tiniest details that you can remember. Writing in a lot of detail can assist you in returning to that place in your mind easier and more efficiently. Some individuals even videotape, sculpt, draw or paint out their descriptions for safekeeping for future use.

- Are there animals or people?

- What do you feel?

- How small or big is your space?

- What colors?

- What surrounds you?

- What is the ultimate backdrop or setting?

- **Visualize positive results** – The main rule of thumb for visualization is imagining situations acted out in positive manners. This involves a heavy amount of thinking happily and setting up a content scene. Imaging positive outcomes are really just a more in-depth version of regular run-of-the-mill positive thinking.

Developing Anxiety Routines

Anxiety routines are any type of daily routine that you use to calm yourself down in stressful situations and that leaves you feeling physical, mental or emotionally distressed. These routines are meant to help you bounce back from the depths of your own thoughts and live a life full of more passion and fulfillment.

This means it is very crucial to choose routines that not only suit you but are healthy, too. Life runs smoother when you have a routine to fulfill those nasty little voices in your head or when you feel like you may make a bad choice because of your anxiety symptoms. Sadly, some people choose unhealthy habitual routines that not only push them back into a negative state but may even provoke symptoms of anxiety and make them worse.

These bad routines could be anything from drug use, both illegal and prescription, large consumption of alcohol or heavy smoking of cigarettes, etc.

You get the picture. Creating an anxiety routine for yourself should not include things that will cause you greater harm in the long run. Honestly, habits like those stated above are only going to make your symptoms worse.

As human beings, we are automatically wired to detect any sort of negative energy that may cause us harm. Anxiety becomes so bad within certain people simply because our bodies do not quite know the difference between stressful triggers that are actually harmless to us versus actual, life-threatening aspects that may be sprung upon us.

Our bodies are made to react to protect ourselves. This is why being mentally prepared for the day that lies ahead of you is so crucial, especially for anxiety sufferers. It is important to back up our thoughts with an extra layer of positivity to promote a sense of safety and well-being. This is much easier said than done, especially when life may not have been a very good friend to you as of late. But being able to mentally develop a positive sense of self is the first step in creating daily routines that help pave your way to a successful life to live and your future.

Routines to Decrease Anxiety

With the right amount of inspiration, the first day or two of adding a new routine to your life can be exciting. You know you are making a positive change that will hopefully help you feel better about yourself and the life you live. However, self-care routines can be a hard thing to manage and utilize on a regular basis once the newness of acting upon it wears off.

Anxiety can leave some sufferers so dismayed by anxious or sad thoughts that they want nothing more than to do away with anything that resonates positive energy. But this is the exact opposite of fighting for yourself and your happiness. Everyone has their bad days and moments and by all means, you are allowed to have and live those. But it is important not to stay tucked away in them for long periods of time.

Developing and executing specific daily routines that you are comfortable with gives those a step by step plan for the day and keeps you prepared for situations or other anxiety triggers from leaping out and mugging you of your happiness. Routines, kind of like exercise, are things we practice daily to keep us in shape, but anxious routines keep our minds in check. You never know when something will catch you off guard, when a person may ask you something that is bothersome or when a debilitating symptom of anxiety will hit you throughout the course of the day. It is better to be prepared than not to be, right?

The Importance of a Balanced Morning Routine

Many functions within routines do them absolutely no good. When the alarm goes off, they tend to hit snooze a few times. When they finally decide to open their eyes, they automatically reach for their phones and look at updates on social media. Many people are already let down by the fact no one messaged them or liked their posts throughout the night.

When their feet finally touch the floor to stand up out of bed, they are already on a path to a negative, self-destructing day. They take a quick shower, down a bowl of cereal and chug a cup of coffee and get to their day job...what is the point?

This lack of routine is non-beneficial. We see our unstructured lives as having no real purpose, which results in a lack of inner peace. We are destroying our happiness without realizing it!

Benefits of a Morning Routine

Creating a morning routine is not only a big part in relieving anxiety, but it also boosts productivity, brings out your inner positivity, helps you to develop and successfully sustain good relationships, as well as being a big reducer of negativities. Morning routines alone have been shown to be the best strategy for reducing stress and relieving those pesky symptoms of anxiety, no matter how long they have resided within you.

Morning routines keep you consciously aware and more grounded throughout the day. In fact, many who were once stubborn and did not want to incorporate a daily routine were eventually surprised at how much better they felt each and every morning. Anxiety levels dropped and confidence and happiness levels substantially rose. A morning routine can literally reduce your anxiety by as much as sixty percent!

Steps to Include in Your Morning Routine

When you **wake up earlier**, you know that you have plenty of time to get up and get ready for your day, which aids in decreased stress levels. If there is adrenaline pumping throughout your body as you rush around to head out the door, it sticks with you for the rest of the day.

Sounds like a waste of time, but **making your bed each morning** is a powerful task that helps you gain the momentum you need to get pumped for the day ahead. For those that suffer from anxiety and depression, making the bed is simple but can make a huge difference because you know you have completed *one* task if not anything else.

Meditation and prayer is a subject with many critics. People view meditation as an act performed only by spiritual individuals. Practicing mindfulness daily has positive side effects that can trigger feel-good hormones in the brains that aid in reducing levels of stress, anxiety and even depression.

Mixing meditation and prayer within your morning routine can be quite vitalizing, giving clarity to your life and your decisions. If you wish to learn more about the power behind the act of prayer, it will be covered in the following chapter The Empowerment of Prayer.

Taking an ice cold shower in the mornings has been proven to provide the human body with a great number of benefits. Cold exposure, also known as cold shower therapy, is nothing new. Our ancestors utilized it as a remedy to treat mental ailments. Showering in cold water provides the body with adequate circulation and tones the skin nicely.

The cold feeling kicks positive responses throughout the body into overdrive. It accelerates the repairing of cells, which reduces inflammation, pain, and speeds up our metabolic processes. The icy waters help lower negative levels that depression and anxiety can hover over us. Standing under the cold water for just a couple minutes can yield you these benefits.

Substitute your breakfast with coffee or tea to bump up energy levels and replace your usual breakfast eats. This is not recommended for absolutely everyone, but if you are trying to find ways to keep hunger away for the first portion of your day, give it a shot!

Learn how to **utilize a journal** to make "morning pages" as part of your routine in the mornings. This is my personal favorite way to "mind dump" any curious or troubling thoughts you had during the previous day and the night before, as well as random ideas that pop into your mind. I write in my journal after taking a shower, since great ideas tend to spring during those few minutes. When you are able to write down all the negative feelings on paper, you can then get through the day with a clearer state of mind.

Practice gratitude by jotting down things you would miss if they were no longer in your life, such as objects, people, etc. into your morning pages.

To start the day on a positive note, **jot down what you are looking forward** to that day. This tells our brains to look up, think up and be bright and helps to relieve anxiety.

Write down your intentions at the beginning of each day, no matter how corny they may sound, such as *"I will choose to be consciously present today."*

Write out important tasks that you wish to achieve during the day to ensure you will feel prepared and have a fulfilling plan. This will ease your mind so that you can develop a clear path of action to achieving that days' goals.

I know I have mentioned writing a lot, but like I said before it is a powerful tool. Every morning our brains are ready to go and on high alert, so it is good to have a well-thought-out plan of action.

Write down at least three to five of the most important tasks that you have to complete. Focus on ones that stress you out just thinking about them. Then, ask yourself the following questions about the tasks you have jotted out so that you can prioritize them accordingly:

- Which tasks will help me inch closer to achieving my main goal?

- What task do I have the most fearful anxious thoughts about?

- Which tasks have the potential to cancel out others if done successfully?

Spend 90 minutes every day working towards accomplishing your priorities. Targeting your main goals during the morning hours help you to get them accomplished productively.

Other Morning Methods to Relieve Anxiety

Play uplifting music to ensure an upbeat, positive mood. Create a playlist to play throughout your morning routine. Make your phone's alarm tone a good song to wake up to. You would be surprised at what a difference this effortless step takes.

Spend time with a pet(s) to help raise your dopamine and serotonin levels, resulting in lessened anxiety and depression. Pets also motivate us to climb out of bed and give us the initiative to take on the day, even when our anxiety tries to get the best of us. Adding them to your morning routine is a bonus for not only you but for your pet's well-being too!

Change your scenery in simple ways; Go outside, take a walk. Visit your favorite café and grab a coffee. Go out with a friend. The longer you dwell in a space that sucks away happiness, the worse you will feel.

Interactions with the outside world can be enough to distract you from your anxious habits. This is another reason routines are so important in aiding anxiety. Avoiding responsibilities can actually damage you mentally more than you realize. It is good to get your attention off the darkness of life that resides inside your head. It only makes your anxiety worse when you sit around and obsess over it.

Coping with anxiety and its symptoms can lead to a life of great discomfort. Having some type of structure in the form of routines can be quite crucial to one's success in living a happy, go-lucky life. The next few chapters will cover other types of routines in detail that can help relieve and maybe even make your symptoms disappear for good! It is all about you to initiate making the change.

Chapter 7: Transforming Your anxiety for a better life

If you are feeling anxious or depressed about your future and are allowing negative thoughts to get the best of you and dampen your motivation for success, then learning to use anxiety to your advantage is a must.

Personally, I have learned to *choose* to view my anxiety has a valuable asset that yields me to lead a more authentic life. I live empathetically, for my anxiety has made me a vulnerable person and thus, helped me deepen my life's relationships.

Having anxiety just means I am not mellow enough to take things for granted in life, therefore, making life a richer experience all the way around. In fact, there are a few inspirational ways that anxiety has helped me to elevate my life:

- Got me actively involved in personal development
- Taught me how to think in the present and act now
- Got me reading more books and discover how it heals the mind
- Started me on tracking my success and not just on failure
- Taught me how to make a positive game out of my life
- Assisted me to take control over my life
- Reconnected me to the habit of learning new things every day
- Showed me the power of meditation and visualization
- Allowed me to see that I am not the only one in my life that suffers from degrees of anxiety
- Has taught me to be a more actively vulnerable person

-

Using Anxiety to Your Advantage

Believe it or not, anxiety can be used for good and can be a powerful force in motivating yourself to achieve your desires. Using stress to add momentum to your life is constructive, instead of allowing it to deconstruct our lives.

Redefining danger

You must learn to see anxiety differently; anxiety, before our brains get a hold of it and dwell, is just a warning sign used for our survival. At this point, you are allowing anxiety to make you feel panicked. But even when that warning sign lights up, it doesn't mean you are in danger. You must save this energy for when you really need to make quick decisions.

Create a list of less to most dangerous to help identify a good spectrum of threats. With that comparison, you will be able to see what "dangerous" situations are safe and which ones are frightening.

Channel your stress properly

Diamonds don't grow from trees; they are coals that turn into something more beautiful through pressure. Channeling stress positively into energy for motivation does take time and can be physically and emotionally draining. But instead of allowing negative thoughts take hold of you and send you down that same spiraling hole of anxiety, look at the situation before you differently; view it as your time to *shine*! When negativity starts to manifest in your mind, challenge those thoughts. When you challenge them, you will find that the negativity in them is totally empty in the first place.

Stop trying to do your best

There are two kinds of people: those that do their best and those that can *do better*. However, those that strive to do their best constantly are the ones that end up emotionally drained than those who do better. Why? Because when you do your best, you are settling. When you strive to *do better,* you accept that you are not doing as good as you know you can. For anxiety sufferers, what they do isn't good enough for them. They either drown in their shortcomings or have learned to take the opportunity to improve themselves.

In those with anxiety, underestimation is a common cognitive distortion. When we tell ourselves that we can do better, we know how to reject our deficiencies and go out of their way to prove themselves wrong.

Chapter 8: Battling anxiety like a true warrior

"The only thing we have to fear is fear itself."

> - *President Theodore Roosevelt*

Marines, SEALs, and Special Forces have no choice but to face life-threatening danger head-on regularly. The fact is, if they do get caught up in fear, they are more likely to lose their lives. While many of us will thankfully never have to face these experiences, why aren't we using the fear-crushing tactics that they use in our own personal lives?

Spend time preparing

If you are worried about a work presentation, stressing over a job interview, or freaking out about the upcoming rap battle that might help you move out of your mom's house, then stop, prepare, and practice instead of sitting around. The key is to lose yourself in the moment, which you to by devoting a ton of energy into preparing for what you are worried about. Spend 75% preparing and 25% for the actual event.

SEALs are able to erase fear by practicing upcoming mission until they feel naturally confident. When the unknown becomes more known to them, they don't have to lie to themselves about the risks, but instead put themselves in a better position to handle the unknown, which develops confidence.

Learn to *manage* fear

One of the best ways to deal with fear is to laugh about it. What? You read that right! Laughter lets you know that things are going to be okay and work out. Don't worry; there is evidence to back this theory up. A study by Stanford University showed that those that were trained to make jokes to respond to negative images. This is a much healthier way to deal with fear. The world is an inevitably twisted place, so seeing the funnier side of things makes it easier to deal with.

Breathe

When your heart is beating from your chest, your joints turn into Jell-O, and sweat is pouring off your face, then the best thing you can do to calm the physical manifestations of fear derived from anxiety is to breathe.

That simple? YES. By just inhaling for four seconds and exhaling for four seconds, SEALs can calm their nervous systems and maintain control of their natural biological responses to fear.

You are essentially bending your body's software to better control the hardware. In other words, you are giving yourself a pretty bomb superpower! Breathing helps the body go from the fight-or-flight response of the sympathetic nervous system to the relaxed response of the parasympathetic nervous system.

Tactical breathing used by Navy SEALS for performance just prior to a tense situation or during a workout:

Breathe through the nose. It's very important to breathe through your nose since breathing through the nose stimulates nerve cells that exist behind sternum near the spine that triggers the parasympathetic nervous system. Anxiety is a sympathetic response and parasympathetic counteracts that. This calms your body, which then calms your mind.

1. Relaxed sitting position and right handle on the belly.
2. Activate the breath by pushing belly out and then inhale deeply for a count of four. Inhale to the belly. This pulls breath deep into the lungs. Exhale through the nose for a count of four, pulling the belly

95

button toward the spine. Repeat this three times.

3. Now breathe in through belly and diaphragm for a count of four, again inhaling into your belly and this time lifting your chest. Again, exhale for a count of four so that your rib cage falls and your belly button pulls toward your spine. Repeat three times.

4. Next, use the same technique, this time inhaling for a count of four through the belly, diaphragm and your chest, with a slight raise of shoulders for inhaling. Exhale for a count of four three the chest, diaphragm, and then the belly. Repeat three times, eventually working your breaths up to eight counts.

Next, box breathing is a technique used by the U.S. Navy SEALS to maintain focus and to calm nervous system after a tense situation, such as combat, an intense workout or anytime the desire is to center and focus.

Trains for diaphragmic breathing or deep breathing. Relaxes the whole system and provides oxygen to the brain to focus better. Improves energy. It can also be used by you to regain your sense of balance, concentration, and relaxation and can be practiced at any time. Use the same technique as tactical breathing but you use a five-count hold between breaths.

1. Get in a relaxed sitting position

2. Inhale deeply through the nose for five seconds

3. Hold the air in your lungs for five seconds

4. Exhale for five seconds, releasing all the air from your lungs

5. Hold your lungs empty for five seconds

6. Repeat for five minutes, or as long as you feel necessary

Don't keep things bottled up

Fear is just like terrible liquor; it sucks when you drink it and has negative effects that last a long time, which is why it is important to deal with it before and after the fact.

Talking about scary experiences helps soldiers locate the meaning behind it all. This communication allows them to process what they have been through positively and helps them to create closer relationships with their mates. Scared? Admit it to a friend. Hearing it out loud can help you pull it out, confront it, and deal with it.

Overpower that inner nagging voice

We are all aware of the inner chatter that occurs in our mind on a daily basis. In fact, our inner voice can be really negative the majority of the time. Wouldn't it be cool to have an inner monologue that reminds us how confident and awesome we are? Wouldn't it be great to have an inner motivational speaker to get us through tough times?

Well, you can. In times of stress, our brains are wired to create self-talk that can increase our feelings of fear. As a soldier, they are expected to fight against their inner self-talk and focus on positive portions of experiences. With practice, they are easily able to ignore or even erase the negativity their brains are throwing at them. So, you can do the same in your own life.

Fear and anxiety thrive when we imagine the worst. We developed imagination to be able to project into the future so we can plan ahead. However, a side effect of being able to imagine possible positive futures is being able to imagine things going wrong. A bit of this is useful; after all, there really might be muggers or loan sharks. But uncontrolled imagination is a testing ground for anxiety and fear that can spoil otherwise happy lives.

Some people misuse their imagination chronically and so suffer much more anxiety than those who either future-project their imaginations constructively or who don't tend to think about the future much at all. Anxious, chronic worriers tend to misuse their imaginations to the extent that upcoming events feel like catastrophes waiting to happen. No wonder whole lives can be blighted by fear and anxiety.

Think of the worst-case scenario

No matter what you are afraid of, you always have the opportunity to avoid it for the rest of your life. However, soldiers don't get that choice. They face similar situations time and time again that scare them. To ensure fear doesn't overrule them, they simulate stressful scenarios and try to experience the emotions with them as well.

Instead of thinking happy thoughts and ignoring what you are afraid of, start looking at the worst things that can possibly happen. When you are able to picture the worst fear and stay within an emotional experience instead of pushing yourself out of it, your mind tends to get over the fear naturally.

Reframe your mindset

Reframe you definition of symptoms. Reframe the symptoms of anxiety - give them a different meaning.   Those sweaty palms, racing heart, and lightheadedness can mean a panic attack or they can mean the most exciting and fun adventure of your life! Your body doesn't know the difference and it is just doing what it does by nature, but you can choose how you define that sudden rush. Don't believe me?

How do you think those adrenaline junkies dives off cliffs, jump motorcycles or swim with sharks? Their definition of what we call fear is definitely different. They still experience the same potent chemicals coursing through their body, but the sensations have a different meaning to them. What you experience as fear, dread and near death can be defined as thrilling, exciting, and aliveness to someone else.

The beautiful thing about consistently and purposely redefining these symptoms is you can actually rewire your brain. This leads us to neuroplasticity.

Neuroplasticity

Neuroplasticity occurs with changes in behavior, thinking, and emotions. With conscious practice, we can alter our neural pathways to move naturally towards our desired emotions, such as being thankful, calm, and happy and away from anger, stress, and panic.

As you choose to respond with positive emotion, you can strengthen the neural pathways to the desired emotions. As you make more neural connections over time to your desired emotion, the pathways to the negative reactions eventually become weaker and scrambled. This even works while using mental rehearsals of the situation and practicing your desired response.

Remember, this can also work in reverse. If you have a habitual response to circumstances, such as being angry in a traffic jam and you repeat these responses over and over in a high state of emotion, you will strengthen the neural pathways towards the emotion of anger in that situation. The masters over the centuries who taught positive thinking and faith may have actually been on to something and now we can prove it scientifically.

Get moving

Exercise is usually associated with weight loss, improved physical health, and a stronger immune system. But the benefits of exercise can expand much more. Exercise is just as important for your mental fitness as it is your physical health. Aerobic activity promotes the release of endorphins that are released in the brain and act as painkillers, which also help to increase a sense of well-being. Endorphins also improve energy levels, provide a better night's sleep, elevate your mood and provide anti-anxiety effects. Exercise also takes your mind off of your worries and breaks the cycle of negative thoughts that contribute to anxiety.

It is recommended to perform 30 minutes or more of exercise five days a week to have a significant impact on anxiety symptoms. You don't need a formal exercise program at the gym to experience these benefits. Light physical activity has been shown to have the same effects, including gardening, housework, washing the car and walking around the block. These can be done in small intervals throughout the day.

It's more important to do some sort of physical activity on a consistent basis than to aim for something that is not sustainable. Be realistic and if you need to start with smaller goals, do so. This is all about taking care of yourself in a way that works for you.

The single, most important natural tool you can use to beat anxiety is regular exercise. It sounds cliché, but the truth is that exercise affects the mind and body in ways that science is still discovering.

There is a reason that anxiety prevalence has grown with our increasingly inactive lifestyles. Jogging every day can make a world of difference in how you deal with stress, how your anxiety symptoms manifest, and how you regulate your mood.

The best methods of exercise to combat anxiety are:

- **Running** releases feel-good hormones that have exponential mental health benefits. It can help you fall asleep faster, improve memory, lower stress levels, and protects against developing depression.

- **Hiking** in a wooded or hilly location has natural calming effects on the brain. Being around plants and Earthly sights helps to reduce anxiety thanks to the chemicals plants emit. Plus, being out in nature is great for your health and memory function.

- **Yoga,** a lot like meditation, has been found to significantly reduce anxiety and other neurotic symptoms that can lead to irritability and depression. It not only strengthens your core but helps you to focus on breathing, which is the key to relaxing the mind and combating anxiety.

Chapter 9: Rediscovering yourself after hurricane anxiety

Those that live with and through the darkness of anxiety can find themselves waking up each day unhappy. Life is short and there comes a time where re-evaluating your life in order to revamp parts of it to ensure your happiness and fulfillment.

We all get lost in life from time to time. We forget old passions we had, give up interest in pursuit of something else, etc. But it is never too late to rediscover what makes you great and what makes you feel truly alive.

When were you the *happiest*?

Take a moment to remember when you were the most content with your life. In high school? College? Before marriage, family, and kids? When you began your family? Started your business? Pursued a new hobby?

No one peaks at the same time or levels in their lives. The key to regaining contentment is not to think of those fond times as "the past", but to figure out how to find that feeling of happiness again where you currently are in your life. How can you re-incorporate those things that brought you joy in the life you are living now?

What makes you *unhappy*?

What makes your blood pressure shoot through the roof? Figuring out the things that push your last buttons is just as important as knowing what helps you keep a positive outlook. When you are able to clearly point out the toxic influences, you will be better able to erase them and develop better, healthier ways of living. We tend to hold onto things from the past that has negative impacts on our current lives. What grudges are you holding onto? These are toxic and are keeping you from being your best self! No matter what it is, from a toxic ex-partner to a job that drains you, cutting these negative influences will allow you ample space to grow in a positive direction.

Write!

When negative thoughts are constantly bouncing around the brain, it can be very easy to become overwhelmed. We tend to forget how much our daily thoughts impact our lives. They take hold of our power, telling us who we are and what are and aren't capable of. We are the only ones that have the power to take action to erase pesky thoughts from inhibiting our success in life.

I have found that organizing thoughts by writing them down makes them more abstract. When you can visualize them on paper, it makes them concrete.

Write out a list of pros and cons, random thoughts that pop up, poetry, grocery lists, anything that comes to mind. All writing can be therapeutic and helps us to rediscover how our voice sounds, which radiates who. I challenge to find yourself again with the power of good old pen and paper.

Learning to Love Yourself Again

To rediscover yourself, you need to learn how to love yourself again for who you are, and all parts of yourself, including your flaws and everything you have endured. There are millions of places that offer up 'good advice' to practice self-love, but they never explain exactly how to do so.

Loving yourself is a vital piece of the puzzle when it comes to positive personal growth. It allows us to fulfill our dreams and create happy and healthy relationships with others too.

Care about yourself as much as you care about others

This sounds almost too simple, but many of us are not selfish enough when it comes to fulfilling our wants and needs. It is hard to remember that you are *not* selfish when it comes to caring about yourself and your wellbeing.

Showing yourself compassion shows those in your life that you are able to take care of yourself. No one can pour from an empty pot, which means you need to take care of yourself in order to take care of others in your life. Treat yourself the way you treat your best friend, with caring, concern, and gentleness, no matter what is happening in your life.

Maintain boundaries

Jot down a list of things you need emotionally, both what is important to you and what upsets you. The list can be made up of anything, from wanting sympathy to being celebrated, to being cared for, etc. Whatever is important to you, no matter how silly it sounds, *Write. It. Down.*

We can often find ourselves smack dab in the middle of the confusing conflict and wonder how we got there in the first place. We ask ourselves how we attracted this situation and the people in it with us. While you still need to take responsibility for your actions, it is also crucial to not fall into a pit of self-blame that can cause stress, but rather really look into what is occurring. Many people lack inner confidence and have no idea what they are worth. This lack can leave us living in a sum-zero equation; we are loved completely or become completely unlovable.

I have found from my psychological studies and personal experiences that there are two very simple questions to help anyone restore healthy boundaries in their life to live a dignified life:

What does this situation negatively represent about yourself? How are you tolerating situations and the behaviors of those around you reinforces your low-worth within you? Those in our lives are a mirror of our own biases, hopes, and fears. *"All anger stems from anger at the self."*

What is your worst fear about saying "no"? Have you ever been left with the thought of you are a bad person because someone's behavior has left you feeling guilty? Well, stop! Challenge that thought by thinking about other situations you have been through. When that happens, the thought that you are a "bad person" falls apart. What matters, in the end, is simple math: people will either *add* or *subtract* to your life.

So, what have you written? The things you write are what you should consider your personal boundaries. When someone ignores something on that list, you should consider it as them crossing boundaries that you have respectively set for yourself. Do not ignore how you feel if this happens, for they are there to tell you what is right from wrong.

Inform others about the boundaries you have set for yourself and be forthcoming with what you will and will not tolerate. When you are assertive with your boundaries, this plays an important part in building a positive self-esteem and allows you many opportunities to reinforce your beliefs, what you cherish, and what you deserve from life.

Do YOU?

Take the time for yourself to establish the things that make you feel good about yourself and about your life as a whole, no matter what it is. Just learn to be aware of how you feel when you go about acting on certain things. For example:

- Are you exhausted by the work you do, but feel thrilled when gardening?
- Are you joyful when reading out loud to your children?
- Do you feel a sense of fulfillment when you write poetry or volunteer in your community?

Once you figure out what makes you feel good about yourself, make those things a priority by implementing them into your every day or weekly schedule. No matter what makes sure you go out and do them! This may mean you have to give up other things to make time for them, but it also means that you may need to re-evaluate your schedule and life more so that you are doing what you honestly enjoy.

To ensure that you are doing these things, there are more than likely going to have to be actions you take to get to those happiness goals, such as saving money to buy supplies to paint, waking up an hour earlier, exercising more, etc.

It is important to realize that you need to do what you need to in order to fulfill your happiness goals. You cannot allow yourself to blame others if you do not fulfill these things. It is time to be a little selfish and fill up your own teapot so that you can fill up the cups of others in your life! This will help you to not only feel better and do better by other people, but it will help you to clear the fog on inconsistent negativity from your life and enable you to truly love yourself and your life once more.

PART III

Chapter 1: Self-Care Is the Best Care

"It is so important to take time for yourself and find clarity. The most important relationship is the one you have with yourself."

-Diane Von Furstenberg

Self-care is any activity that we deliberately do to improve our own well-being, whether it is physical, emotional, mental, or spiritual. The importance of taking care of one's self cannot be denied, as even health care training focuses on making sure healthcare workers are caring for themselves. If you do not take care of yourself, eventually, every other aspect o your life will fall apart, including your ability to help others.

This is a very simple concept, yet it is highly overlooked in the grand scheme of things. People lack the tendency to look after themselves and put their needs before anyone else. Good self-care is essential to improving our mood and reducing our anxiety levels. It will do wonders for reducing exhaustion and burnout, which is very common in our fast-paced world. It will also lead to positive improvements in our relationships.

One thing to note is that self-care does not mean forcing ourselves to do something we don't like, no matter how enjoyable it is to other people. For example, if your friends are forcing you to go to a party you rather not attend, then giving in is not taking care of yourself. If you would rather stay in and watch a movie, then that's what you should do, and it will be better for your well-being.

How Does Self-Care Work

It is difficult to pinpoint exactly what self-care is, as it is personal for everybody. Some people love to pamper themselves by going to the spa, while others enjoy physical activities like hiking, biking, or swimming. Some individuals take up art or other hobbies, like writing or playing a musical instrument. These activities are all different but will have the same type of benefits for the individuals engaging in them.

The main factor to consider when engaging in self-care is to determine if you enjoy the activity in question. If not, then it's time to move on. Self-care is an active choice that you actually have to plan out. It is time you set aside for yourself to make sure all of your needs are met. If you use a planner of any sort, make sure to dedicate some space for your particular self-care activities. Also, let people who need to know about your plans so you can become more committed. Pay special attention to how you feel afterward. The objective of any self-care activity is to make yourself feel better. If this is not happening, then it's time to change the activity.

While self-care, as a whole, is individualized, there is a basic checklist to consider.

- Create a list of things you absolutely don't want to do during the self-care process. For instance, not checking emails, not answering the phone, avoiding activities you don't enjoy, or not going to specific gatherings, like a house party.

- Eat nutritious and healthy meals most of the time, while indulging once in a while.

- Get the proper amount of sleep according to your needs.

- Avoid too many negative things, like news or social media.

- Exercise regularly.

- Spend appropriate time with your loved ones. These are the people you genuinely enjoy and not forced relationships.

- Look for opportunities to enjoy yourself and laugh.

- Do at least one relaxing activity a day, like taking a bath, going for a walk, or cooking a meal.

Self-care is extremely important and should not be an anomaly in your life.

How Does Self-Care Improve Self-Esteem and Self-Confidence?

To bring everything full circle, self-care plays a major role in improving self-esteem and self-confidence. It is easy to see how taking care of yourself will also make you feel better about yourself overall. All of these are actually inter-related, and a lack of one showcases a lack of the other. While caring for yourself also improves your self-esteem and self-confidence, not having self-esteem or self-confidence also leads to a lack of self-care. Basically, you believe that you are not good enough to be taken care of.

People with high self-esteem and self-confidence value themselves as much as they value others, and have no issues with making sure they're taken care of. They realize that it does not make them selfish or inconsiderate to think in this manner. Even if other people try to make them feel that way, a self-confident person will just brush off the criticism. An important thing to note is that when you take care of yourself, it does not mean you don't care about other people. It simply means you have enough self-love to not place yourself on the backburner.

Many people work so hard to try and please everyone else. This is one of the telltale signs of low self-esteem. While they're busy worried about other peoples' needs, their own get neglected, which will wear them down over time. The more they're unable to please someone, the harder they will try. What people in this situation don't realize is that some people are impossible to please, and it is not their responsibility to please them. That is up to the individual.

Poor self-care will eventually lead to poor self-image. It is possible that a person already has this initially. Self-care includes taking care of your hygienic and grooming needs. If you don't take the time to make yourself look good, this will significantly impact the value you place on yourself. When you are t work, among your friends, or just walking around town, not feeling like you look good will ultimately make you feel like you don't belong anywhere. Your confidence levels will plummet due to this.

Your health is another aspect to consider. Poor self-care means bad sleeping habits, unhealthy diets, lack of exercise, and more self-destructive behaviors. Your poor health practices can result in chronic illnesses down the line, like heart disease or diabetes. Once again, diminished health will lead to reduced self-confidence and self-esteem. Ask yourself now if putting other people ahead of you is worth it? I've got some news for you. The people who demand the most from you are probably looking out for themselves first.

The less a person takes care of themselves, the more their self-esteem and self-confidence will decline. It turns into a vicious downward cycle. This is why it is important to focus on all of these areas equally. When you find yourself neglecting your own self-care practices, it is time to shift your direction and bring your attention back to your needs. Ignoring your needs will ultimately lead to your fall. We will discuss specific practices and techniques for improving self-care in the next chapter.

Chapter 2:

What Does Good Self-Care Look Like?

Good Self-Care Practices

The following are some ways that good self-care will look like. If you find yourself having these qualities, then you are on the right path.

Taking Responsibility for Your Happiness

When you engage in self-care, it is truly self-care. This means you only rely on yourself, and nobody else, to make sure your needs are met. You realize that your happiness is no one else's responsibility but your own. You alone have the ability to control your outcomes. As a result of this independence, you will develop the skills and attitude you need to care for your own physical, mental, emotional, and spiritual well-being.

You Become Assertive With Others

People often take assertiveness for rudeness. This is not true, but if people believe that standing firm for what you want is rude, then that's their problem. Once you reach a certain mindset where self-care is important to you, then you will be unapologetically assertive. This means you have the ability to say "no" with confidence and stand by it. "No" is a complete sentence, and people will realize that quickly when they hear it from you.

You Treat Yourself As You Would a Close Friend

It's interesting how we believe that other people deserve better treatment from us than we do ourselves. We have a tendency to put our best friends in front of us, no matter how detrimental it is to our lives. This behavior stops once we engage in proper self-care. At this point, you will treat yourself as good as, or even better, than you treat your most beloved friends.

You Are Not Afraid to Ask for What You Want

Once you learn to take care of yourself, you also see your value increase within your mind. This means having an understanding that your voice, opinion, and needs matter, just like anybody with high self-esteem and self-confidence, would. As a result, you will not be afraid to ask for what you want, even if you might not get it.

Your Life Is Set Around Your Own Values

Once you practice self-care, you learn to check in with yourself before making important decisions. You always make sure the choices you are about to make line up with your purpose and values. If they go against them, then it's not a path you choose. This goes for the career you choose, where you decide to live, and the relationships you maintain in your life.

While all of the traits are focused on self, but it will lead to better relationships with other people too. When you practice self-care, you are in a better state in every aspect of your being. This gives you the ability to take care of and help those you need you, as well. Self-care is not an option, but a necessity, and it must never be ignored. Taking care of yourself is not selfish, no matter what anybody tells you. If someone tries to make you feel guilty over this matter, then consider distancing or removing them from your life. You are not obligated to maintain relationships with people.

Chapter 3: Demanding Your Own Self-Care

We went over the importance of self-care, and now we will focus on making it a reality in your life. If you want self-care to occur, you must be willing to demand it. The world is full of people who expect you to be at there beck-and-call every moment of the day. Some of these individuals are those who are closest to us, like friends or family members. This can make it harder to make our demands heard, but there is no way around it. Taking care of yourself is not an idea you can budge on. It is extremely important. We will go over several ways to maintain your ability for self-care in your life and provide detailed action steps to help you progress in this area.

Setting Healthy Boundaries

One of the biggest obstacles to self-care is other people who surround you. These are the true selfish individuals, whether they realize it or not, who believe they can barge in on your life and deserve all of your attention. They will take advantage of you, and if you are not careful, they will completely gain control of your emotions, and even your life. For proper self-care to occur, you must set firm and healthy boundaries with people. The following are steps that need to become mainstays in your life.

Identify and Name Your Limits

You must understand what your emotional, physical, mental, and spiritual limits are. If you do not know, then you will never be able to set real boundaries with people. Determine what behaviors you can tolerate and accept, and then consider what makes you feel uncomfortable. Identifying and separating these traits will help us determine our lines.

Stay Tuned Into Your Feelings

Two major emotions that are red flags that indicate a person is crossing a barrier are resentment or discomfort. Whenever you are having these feelings, it is important to determine why. Resentment generally comes from people taking advantage of us or feelings of being unappreciated. In this instance, we are likely pushing ourselves beyond our limits because we feel guilty. Guilt-trips is a weapon that many people use to get their way. It is important to recognize when someone is trying to make you feel guilty because they are way overstepping their boundaries. Resentment could also be due to someone imposing their own views or values onto us. When someone makes you feel uncomfortable, that is another indication of a boundary crossed. Stay in tune with both of these emotions.

Don't Be Afraid of Being Direct

With some people, setting boundaries is easy because they have a similar communication style. They can simply read your cues and back off when needed. For other individuals, a more direct approach is needed. Some people just don't get the hint that they've crossed a line. You must communicate to them in a firm way that they have crossed your limits, and you need some space. A respectful person will honor your wishes without hesitation. If they don't, then that's on them. Your personal space is more important than their feelings.

Give Yourself Permission to Set Boundaries

The potential downfalls to personal limits are fear, self-doubt, and guilt. We may fear the other person's response when we set strong boundaries. Also, we may feel guilty if they become emotional about it. We may even have self-doubt on whether we can maintain these limits in the long run. Many individuals have the mindset that in order to be a good daughter, son, parent, or friend, etc., we have to say "yes" all the time. They often wonder if they deserve to have boundaries and limits with those closest to them. The answer is, yes, you do. You need to give yourself permission to set limits with people because they are essential to maintaining healthy relationships too. Boundaries are also a sign of self-respect. Never feel bad for respecting yourself.

Consider Your Past and Present

Determine what roles you have played throughout your life in the various relationships you have had. Were you the one who was always the caretaker? If so, then your natural tendency may be to put others before yourself. Also, think about your relationships now. Are you the one always taking care of things, or is it a reciprocal relationship? For example, are you always the one making plans, buying gifts, having dinner parties, and being responsible for all of the important aspects of the relationships? If this is the case, then tuning into your needs is especially important here. If you are okay with the dynamics of the relationship, then that's fine. I can't tell you how to feel. However, if you feel anger and resentment over this, then it's time to let your feeling be known, unapologetically.

Be Assertive

Once again, this does not mean being rude, even though some people will interpret it that way. Being assertive simply means being firm, which is important when reminding someone about your boundaries. Creating boundaries alone is not enough. You also have to stand by them and let people know immediately if they've crossed them. Let the person know in a respectful but strong tone that you are uncomfortable with where they're going, and they need to give you some space. Assertive communication is a necessity.

Start Small

Setting boundaries is a skill that takes a while to develop, especially if it's something you've never done before. Therefore, start with a small boundary, like no phone calls after a certain time at night. Make sure to follow through;

otherwise, the boundary is worthless. From here, make larger boundaries based on your comfort level.

Eliminating Toxicity and Not Caring About Losing Friends

If you plan on making self-care a priority in your life, I think that's great, and so should you. However, some people will have a problem with this. People don't always like it when their friends, family members, or acquaintances, etc., put themselves at the forefront of their lives. Once again, that is their problem, not yours. What is your problem, though, is distancing or even eliminating these individuals from your life. We will go over that in this section because part of self-care is eliminating toxicity from your life and not feeling bad about it.

Don't Expect People to Change

While everyone deserves a chance to redeem themselves, there comes the point where we must accept that people cannot change by force. They have to find it within themselves to make this change, and it is not our responsibility to do so. You may yearn to be the one who changes them, but it's usually a hopeless project. Toxic individuals are motivated by their problems. They use them to get the attention they need. Stop being the one to give it to them.

Establish and Maintain Boundaries

I already went in-depth on this, so I won't revisit it too much here. Just know that toxic people will push you to work harder and harder for them, while you completely ignore your own needs. This is exhausting and unacceptable. Create the boundaries you need with these individuals based on your own limits.

Don't Keep Falling for Crisis Situations

Toxic people will make you feel like they need you always because they are constantly in a crisis situation of some sort. It is a neverending cycle. When a person is in a perpetual crisis, it is of their own doing. They often create drama purposely to get extra attention. You may feel guilty for ignoring them, but remember that their being manipulative and not totally genuine.

I am not saying that you can't ever help someone who is going through a hard time. Of course, you can. Just don't start believing that you're responsible for their success or failure.

Focus on the Solution

Toxic individuals will give you a lot to be angry and sad about. If you focus on this, then you will just become miserable. You must focus on the solution, which, in this case, is removing drama and toxicity from your life. Recognize the fact that you will have less emotional stress once you remove this person from your life. If you let them, they will suck away all of your energy.

Accept Your Own Difficulties and Weaknesses

A toxic person will know how to exploit your weaknesses and use them against you. For example, if you are easy to guilt-trip, they will have you feel guilty every time you pull away from them. If you get to know yourself better and recognize these weaknesses, then you can better manage them and protect yourself. This goes along with creating self-awareness, which we discussed in chapter two. When you accept your weaknesses, you can work on fixing them and balance them with your strengths.

They Won't Go Easily

Recognize that a toxic individual may resist being removed from your life. Actually, if they don't resist, I will be pleasantly surprised. They may throw tantrums, but this is because they can't control or manipulate you anymore. They will even increase their previous tactics with more intensity. It is a trap, and you must not fall for it. Stay firm in your desire to leave and keep pushing forward. If they suck you back in, good luck trying to get out again.

Choose Your Battles Carefully

Fighting with a toxic person is exhausting and usually not worth it. You do not need to engage in every battle with them. They are just trying to instigate you.

Surround Yourself With Healthy relationships

Once you have removed a toxic person, or persons, from your life, then avoid falling into the trap with someone else. Fill your circle with happy and healthy relationships, so there is no room for any toxicity. Always remember the signs of a toxic person, so you can avoid them wholeheartedly in the future.

How to Focus on Self-Care

Now that we have worked to set boundaries and eliminate toxic people from our lives, it is time to focus on ourselves and the self-care we provide. The following are some self-care tips, according to psychologist, Dr. Tchiki Davis, Ph.D.

Pay Attention to Your Sleep

Sleep is an essential part of taking care of yourself. You must make it part of your routine because it will play a huge role in your emotional and physical well-being. There are many things that can wreak havoc on your sleep patterns, like stress, poor diet, watching television, or looking at your phone as you're trying to fall asleep. Think about your night routine. Are you eating right before bed or taking in a lot of sugar and caffeine? Are you working nonstop right up until bedtime? Have you given yourself some time to wind down before going to sleep? All of these factors are important to consider, as they will affect your sleep patterns. If you can, put away any phones, tablets, and turn off the television at least 30 minutes before you plan on going to bed.

Take Care of Your Gut

We often neglect our digestive tract, but it plays a major role in our health and overall well-being. When our gut is not working well, it makes us feel sluggish, bloated, and nonproductive. Pay attention to the food you eat as it will determine the health of your gut. It is best to avoid food with excess salt, sugar, cholesterol, or unhealthy fats. Stick to foods that are high in fiber, protein, healthy fats, and complex carbs. Some good options are whole grains, nuts, lean meats, fruits and vegetables, beans, and fish.

Exercise and Physical Activity Is Essential

Regular exercise is great for both physical and mental health. The physical benefits are obvious. However, many people do not realize that exercise will help the body release certain hormones like endorphins and serotonin. These are often called feel-good hormones because they play a major role in affecting our mood in a positive way. The release of these hormones will give us energy too, which will make us want to exercise more. Once exercise becomes a habit, it will be hard to break. Decide for yourself what your exercise routine will be, whether it's going to the gym, walking around the neighborhood, or playing a game of tennis.

Consider a Mediterranean Diet

While this is not a dietary book, the Mediterranean diet is considered the healthiest diet in the world because of its extreme health benefits. The food groups and ingredients that are used will increase energy, brain function, and has amazing benefits like heart and digestive tract health. The food also does not lack flavor, which shatters the myth that healthy food does not taste good.

Take a Self-Care Trip

Even if you are not much of a traveler, getting away once in a while can do wonders for your mental health. So often, our environment will make us feel stressed out, and it's good to remove ourselves from it for a couple of days. You do not have to take a trip abroad here. Of course, that is certainly an option. A simple weekend trip is perfectly fine. Just get yourself out of your normal routine and be by yourself for a while.

Get Outside

Nature and sunlight can be great medicines. It can help you reduce stress or worry, and has many great health benefits. Doing some physical activity outside, like hiking or gardening, are also great options.

Bring a Pet Into Your Life

Pets can bring you a lot of joy, and the responsibility they come with can boost your self-confidence by having to care for another living creature. Dogs are especially great at helping to reduce stress and anxiety. Animal therapy has been used to help people suffering from disorders lie PTSD, as well.

Get Yourself Organized

Organizing your life and doing some decluttering can do wonders for your mental and emotional health. Decide what area of your life needs to be organized. Do you need to clear your desk, clean out the fridge, or declutter your closet? Do you need to get a calendar or planner and schedule your life better? Whatever you can do to get yourself more organized, do it. Being organized allows you to know how to take better care of yourself.

Cook Yourself Meals At Home

People often neglect the benefits of a good home-cooked meal. They opt, instead, for fast-food or microwave dinners. These types of meals will make you full but will lack in essential nutrients that your body needs. Cooking nutritious meals at home will allow you to use the correct ingredients, so you can feel full and satisfied. Cooking alone can also be great therapy for people.

Read Regularly

Self-help books are a great read. However, do not limit yourself to these. You can also read books on subjects that you find fascinating or books that simply provide entertainment.

Schedule Your Self-Care Time

Just like you would write down an appointment time in your planner, also block out specific times for self-care activities. Stick to this schedule religiously, unless a true emergency comes up. This means that if a friend calls you to go out, you should respectfully decline their request and focus on yourself.

Chapter 4: How to Be Happy Being Alone

The final section of this book will focus on being alone and how to be happy about it. When you start engaging in self-care, you will also be spending much more time by yourself. A lot of people have a hard time dealing with this concept, especially if they're used to being around people all the time. However, for proper self-care, you have to be okay with being alone once in a while.

Accept Some Alone Time

The following are some tips to help you become happy with being alone. Soon, you will realize that your own company is the best kind.

Do Not Compare Yourself to Others

We are referring to your social life here. Do not compare to others, and do not feel like you must live as others do. If you do this, you may become jealous of a person's social circle or lifestyle. It is better to focus on yourself and what makes you happy. If you plan on spending significant time alone, then you cannot pay attention to what other people are doing.

Step Away From Social Media

If strolling through your social media page makes you feel left out, then take a step back and put it away for a while. During self-care moments, you are the focus, not what is happening with others online. Also, what people post on their pages is not always true. Many individuals have been known to exaggerate, or even flat-out lie on social media platforms. You may be feeling jealous or left out for no reason. Try banning yourself from social media for 24-48 hours, and see how it makes you feel.

Take a Break From Your Phone

Avoid making or receiving calls. Let the important people in your life know that you will be away from your phone for a while, so they don't worry. When you are alone, really try to be alone.

Allow Time for Your Mind to Wander

If you feel unusual about doing nothing, it is probably because you have not allowed yourself to be in this position for a while. Carve out a small amount of time where you stay away from TV, music, the internet, and even books. Use this time to just sit quietly with your thoughts. Find a comfortable spot to sit or lie down, then just let your mind wander and see where it takes you. This may seem strange the first time, but with practice, you will get used to the new freedom.

Take Yourself on a Date

You don't need to be with someone else to enjoy a night out on the town. Take a self-date and enjoy your own company for a while. Go to a movie by yourself, stop by a nice restaurant, or just go do an activity you enjoy. If you are not used to hanging out alone, give it some time and you will become more comfortable with it. Take yourself on that solo date.

Exercise

We have mentioned exercise and physical activity a lot, but that's because it has so many great benefits related to self-care. Exercising will uplift your mood, and make it more enjoyable to be by yourself. Those feel-good hormones will provide a lot of benefits during these times.

Take Advantage of the Perks of Being Alone

Some people have spent so much time with other people that they've forgotten the perks of being alone. There are many to consider. First of all, you do not have to ask anyone's permission to do anything; you will have more personal space, can enjoy the activities you want to do, and don't have to worry about upsetting anyone. If you want, you can even have a solo dance party in your living room, Tom Cruise style. There are many advantages to being alone, so use them.

Find a Creative Outlet

It is beneficial to use some of your alone time to work on something creative. This can be painting, sculpting, music, writing, or any other creative endeavors. In fact, you can get out the watercolors and start fingerpainting. Creativity will bring a lot of joy into your life. It will make you happier about being alone.

Take Time to Self-Reflect

Being alone will give you the opportunity to self-reflect on your life. You won't care so much about being alone when you are coming up with important answers to your life.

Make Plans for Your Future

Planning out your life for five or ten years down the line will give you something important to do, and something to look forward to. Alone time is the perfect opportunity to determine these plans.

Make Plans for Solo Outings

Plan your solo outings based on what you like to do, whether it's a farmer's market, hiking, riding your bike, or going camping alone. Mak plans that will excite you, and you will be taking care of yourself while also being okay alone.

There are numerous topics that we went over in this chapter, but they all relate back to one theme: Self-care. Always remember that to take proper care of yourself, you must consider the following ideas:

- Setting Boundaries
- Avoiding and ridding yourself of toxic people
- Focus on yourself and your needs
- Be okay with being alone

Focus on these areas, and you will be demanding your own self-care without ever apologizing for it.

PART IV

Chapter 1: What is CBT?

None of us have control over every aspect of our lives. Therefore, we all must play the hands we are dealt as we navigate through life. Unfortunately, many of the circumstances we have to deal with are unpleasant and can leave us with lasting scars that can start a domino effect of negative thoughts that seem to never end.

It is important to understand that our ability to control many of the elements in our lives is out of our hands; we can't even control the thoughts that seem to flow endlessly through our minds. Still, this does not mean that we are completely helpless. While much of these things happen against our will, there are many things we can do to change the situations we face. At the very least, we can control how we respond to the external events and factors we deal with from day to day. We have the ability to control our reactions to events, thoughts, and internal beliefs about what is happening to us.

This adjusted kind of thinking is at the heart of CBT. It is a research-based approach to a treatment that will address a wide variety of mood and anxiety disorders. A fundamental belief behind CBT is that after experiencing certain situations, certain thoughts are developed in the mind. These thoughts lead to a variety of different feelings (many unpleasant), which can trigger negative reactions. Since feelings are not that easy to change, the concentration of the therapy is on challenging the thoughts that trigger those feelings and once you can control your feelings, you will be able to control your actions. As you develop these new skills, you will be able to manage your life better, which by extension, will allow you to build up a more positive view of the world, and thus have an improved pattern of behavior.

So, rather than pouring out your past to a therapist, opening up painful wounds of the past, and examining every minute detail of them, you and your therapist will work together to discuss the problems you are facing today, set a series of goals, and then apply different strategies and exercises you can apply to help you achieve them.

The Science Behind It

Unlike psychoanalysis, a common form of therapy developed by Sigmund Freud, where treatment is based on early life experiences and uncovering hidden memories that may have been buried, CBT takes an entirely different approach in healing the mind. In CBT, the problems are the foundation for the treatment.

In the early part of the 20th century when psychoanalysis was the accepted form of treatment, you would have spent an endless number of sessions talking about your past. The psychoanalyst would likely interrupt your dialogue with occasional questions about what you might think this image or that person meant, forcing you to think deeper about your reaction to certain events, people, and influences in your life. His goal would have been to get you to explore hidden messages stashed somewhere in your psyche.

At some point, the treatment would gradually take effect and your feelings would start to experience a change. This form of treatment, while effective, would often require a long-term commitment, which could take years to complete, if ever.

About the middle of the 20th century, we began to understand better how the brain worked. Initial research into the function of this organ started focusing on the more recent scientific discoveries relating to both animal behavior and then later in the field of metacognition.

As scientific research progressed over the last century, they have been able to develop a better understanding of learning, behavior, and cognition (our thoughts); it was a natural progression from Freud's form of therapy to what we use now. First, experimenters began to recognize that even animals could associate two separate events together. For example, an experimenter would ring a bell and then give food to a dog. After this action was repeated several times, the dog would automatically associate the bell with food. It was apparent that the dog understood that the sound of the bell meant food.

The next progression was the discovery that helped us understand how human behavior developed. Scientists wanted to understand what would make a person more likely to do one thing and less likely to do another. It was quickly understood that if you punish someone for an action (giving them an unpleasant result), then they would cease the action. The opposite was true with a reward system. If a reward was given, the individual would then be encouraged to continue the action.

This knowledge was quickly applied to mental health where they could now focus their attention on treating the behavior of a patient rather than rehashing all of its past experiences. The patients that are most benefited from this type of therapy are, in a sense, stuck in a certain pattern of behavior. The trigger for that behavior may have happened in his or her childhood or it may have happened in the past few months. The time of the trigger or the real nature of it is not as important as addressing the present state of affairs. The therapy, therefore, is focused on changing that behavior so that he can get out of his rut and start living his life again.

The next evolution of CBT was developed much later in the 60s and 70s. The focus then was on identifying what was really triggering that behavior. It was determined that it was the power of the thoughts and their effect on emotions, which in turn, was triggering the actions. Psychiatrists recognized that to understand how a person feels, they must first understand what a person was

131

really thinking. If a person is struggling with anxiety, then chances are their thoughts were full of thoughts of danger or risk.

Up until that point, they had recognized the cause and effect scenario that was playing out in a person's mind. For example, someone who is afraid of elevators would see the elevator and automatically feel fear.

What they realized later was that there was one missing element that needed to be understood. It wasn't the elevator that was causing the fear in the person, but it was their mind's interpretation of what that elevator actually meant. This goes back to the original premise that what a person thinks is what dictates his emotions and his behavior.

However, we all know that what we think and believe is not always accurate. According to his book *Healing the Addicted Brain*, Dr. Harold Urschel explains that once you begin to analyze your thoughts, you will inevitably find inaccuracies in your reasoning. These inaccuracies tend to reappear over and over again in your mind until corrected. In other words, all of us have distorted thinking and need to be aware of them. In fact, just the simple act of recognizing and acknowledging them will automatically make it easier to change your thought process and help you to replace them with healthier thoughts.

So, if one can get inside the thought process and find the flaw, correcting certain behaviors could be addressed simply by correcting the wrong thoughts that were playing out in their mind at the time. This means that if a person was struggling with irrational thoughts, these could be replaced with more realistic beliefs through a process of challenging them and arming them with a new way of thinking. Analysts were no longer focused on finding the root cause of a problem and could now focus on changing the thoughts that trigger unwanted behaviors.

Through CBT, analysts could help their patients by giving them a set of skills that could be learned, practiced, and through a regular application on their own, could work independently to address their issues.

How it Works

As you read these words, the whole process sounds relatively simple. At first glance, you might have even wondered why a person would need a therapist to figure this out, and you'd be right. But, for those who are stuck in that endless loop of unwanted behavior, it still remains a real challenge.

It is a huge step from Freudian therapy to CBT. A person has to first come to the understanding that three core elements of our human makeup are completely interconnected: our thoughts, feelings, and behaviors. It is literally impossible to change one without changing either of the other two.

This concept can be illustrated simply. If you are struggling with feelings of anxiety, it is usually because your mind is overwhelmed with thoughts of dangers that you want to avoid. However, if your thoughts of danger are distorted, then your reaction to those thoughts will be strange, out of the ordinary, and even extreme. It is only a short step from a fear of danger to trigger our fight-or-flight response, which will either cause us to avoid the situation altogether or to take an aggressive stance.

The Basic Principles of CBT: In order for CBT to be effective, there has to be a good relationship between the therapist and the client. At the very least, there must be a mutual respect for each other and it is extremely important for the therapist to get a good understanding of how the client sees things.

From this area of mutual respect, the foundation for treatment can be laid. After that, there are several other basic principles that must be followed:

- CBT is not an open-ended therapy session – it has a time limit. In most cases, the time with a therapist runs only 10-15 sessions. This puts a slight pressure on the client to not procrastinate in getting started with the specific steps the therapist will give him as homework. He is less likely to put it off until a more convenient time.

- CBT is based on more than a century of research studies. From the beginning, a therapist can give a pretty reasonable estimate as to how long a program can run given the client's unique mental state of mind, and how much of a benefit he can expect to achieve in that time period. As they work together through the sessions, it will be easy to see which parts of the program are working well and which ones are not and make adjustments accordingly.

- CBT always has a very specific objective for the client. It is not about looking at the past but is more about achieving a specific goal. You can't make progress if you don't have a direction to go in, and it won't take long before you will see evidence that the program is helping you to get to the behavior you want to display.

- CBT is a team effort. The therapist doesn't "fix" you. You work together to address and discuss out a certain issue. Each party in the team has something to contribute; the specialist understands just how CBT works, and you (the client) understand how you work. Bringing the two together, as a team, allows both to tailor a treatment that will address the specific needs of the client.

- CBT is well-organized. CBT sessions are not hours of aimless ramblings with a therapist. Instead, they have structured in such a way that the patient knows exactly what his objectives are and the steps they are going to take to get there. The first sessions are dedicated to creating a roadmap outlining every step in the treatment plan. Throughout the program, both the therapist and patient can check to see if they are still on course or if adjustments are needed.

- CBT is about the present. While CBT looks at past events in a patient's life, its primary focus is on what can be done today to fix the problem. It stresses the importance of finding ways to change thoughts and behaviors today so that there can be immediate relief.

- CBT involves action. Both the therapist and the patient are fully engaged in the process. Without a commitment from both parties, it won't be successful. From the very beginning, it requires both to be fully involved with each stage of the treatment.

- CBT focuses on skills. Patients go through each therapy session learning different skills they can continue to use once the session is over. These skills teach you how to identify the mind games you play with yourself, the self-sabotaging strategies you use, and teach you how to stop those bad habits in their tracks and choose healthier and more productive options.

- CBT stresses practice. You have 168 hours in a week and can count on only one hour of time with your therapist. So, in order to get the most out of each session, it is important that you practice each of the strategies learned in your session on your own. The more work is done in between sessions the faster the progress will be.

Changes Thought Patterns and Belief Systems

Since Cognitive Behavioral Therapy is based on the evidence that our *perceptions* of the situations in our lives dictate how we feel emotionally, our perceptions of the world are, therefore, the direct result of what we think is really happening or will happen. These are the elements of our lives that need to be adjusted.

For example, an individual may find something in this book and think it is exactly what he is looking for. Because he *believes* it is beneficial for him, he then feels good and perhaps even relieved to have found the solution to his problem. However, another person may read the same information and feel entirely different. He may believe that it isn't the right solution for him or that following the exercises are beyond the scope of his ability. As a result, he will feel disappointed and maybe even discouraged at not finding the answer to his problem.

In theory, it is not the experience that causes people to feel the way they do, but it is their perception of the situation or their thoughts about the experience that needs to be modified. We all understand that when a person is under stress, their viewpoint of a situation is often extreme, inaccurate, and unrealistic, so if it is the perception of an experience that triggers negative habits, then this is the area that needs to be focused on.

With CBT, people are helped to identify those negative thoughts, give an honest and realistic appraisal of them, and then learn strategies to help them to readjust their distorted thinking. Once they are able to think more realistically, they will begin to see things differently and it will be easier for them to adjust their behaviors. The therapy works within a narrow focus of solving their immediate problems and making behavioral changes.

Its Purpose – Who it Can Help

Of course, CBT is not a catch-all for all psychological disorders. It has proven to be most effective for the treatment of anxiety, depression, and other forms of mood disorders including obsessive-compulsive disorder, bipolar, and PTSD. While the National Institute for Health and Care Excellence (NICE) specifically recommends CBT for the treatment of anxiety and depression, there are many more mental health issues that it can be very effective with.

Because of its unique flexibility, the therapy can easily be adapted to a wide range of needs. There is a whole list of psychological issues that can be benefited by it including:

- ADD/ADHD
- Alcohol abuse
- Anger management
- Anxiety
- Bipolar disorder
- Borderline personality disorder
- Chronic fatigue syndrome
- Chronic pain
- Depression
- Drug abuse
- Eating disorders
- Facial tics
- Insomnia
- Obsessive-compulsive disorder
- Phobias
- Post-traumatic stress disorder
- Psychosis
- Relationship problems (individual or couple's therapy)
- Schizophrenia

In most cases, it can be a very effective form of treatment without the use of medication, but in extreme cases, where the symptoms a patient is experiencing are severe, a doctor may suggest the use of medications to make it easier to get into a mental state where patients can effectively apply the strategies suggested as they go through the program.

How it Works on Anxiety and Depression

When dealing with anxiety disorders, one must first come to understand the true nature of anxiety. While unpleasant in many ways, a certain level of anxiety is necessary for life. Without it, we would find ourselves in an even worse predicament. Consider all the ways a healthy sense of anxiety can be of benefit.

Both anxiety and fear are natural forms of emotions. They serve as your body's personal alarm system and can occur as a warning sign that there may be some kind of risk or harm present. Fear, a heightened sense of anxiety, appears when a person is literally faced with a dangerous situation. Anxiety occurs when they "expect" that something unpleasant is about to happen.

A good example of this is taking a ride on a roller coaster. The feeling you get as the car is slowly pulled up that first big hill. You are in anticipation of what you know is about to happen as soon as you reach the top. Fear is the feeling you get when you are plummeting down the hill.

Both emotions are warnings and can trigger all sorts of bodily sensations. They tap into our flight-or-fight response so that we can quickly respond to those warnings, allowing us to flee, freeze, or fight. These instinctive emotions have been a part of us for as long as the human race has existed. It is a highly developed system that allows us to react quickly without having to put forth a lot of effort. They make it possible for us to have an automatic response.

The problem with these emotions is evident when they become overactive. It is natural for humans to have a very active imagination that allows our minds to create certain scenarios that we may encounter. For example, you may be anticipating how a certain job interview will play out. Your mind may conjure up something good or something very bad, both could result in anxiety even though there is no assurance that what you imagined will actually happen. This is evidence that our internal alarm system can be triggered even when there is no real threat to deal with.

The natural progression is that if our automatic thoughts are negative, we will respond accordingly. As a result, if we have conjured up images of a bad interview, our reactions could be so strong that we can take some very negative actions that could harm us in some way. For example, we might refuse to show up for the interview, we might choose to apply for a job that we find less challenging or risky, or we might become so flustered that we blow the interview altogether causing our worst fears to come true. These choices could actually have a very negative effect on our lives causing us even more harm in the future.

Anxiety and depressive disorders can appear in a variety of forms. Episodes may be occasional or they may be constant. If these automatic thoughts are not addressed, they will only become more sensitive starting a spiral effect that will send a person deeper and deeper into a level of anxiety that will be even more difficult to get out of.

CBT is most effective because it works to correct those automatic thoughts. Those spontaneous thoughts we all have that spring to mind without prompting. Automatic thoughts start before we are born and will continue unabated until we take our last breath. It is our brain's way of processing the millions of bits of information it is constantly receiving from our five senses: sight, sound, smell, taste, and touch. If the brain receives any input from these sources under a stressful situation, it can create unfounded assumptions about a given situation or possible outcome. These negative assumptions create an unhealthy internal dialog that could build up to a point that it prevents an individual from progressing when faced with similar circumstances. Unless this internal dialog is corrected, the resulting negative emotions or behavior could take control causing the person to be paralyzed to the point of inaction or to exercise complete avoidance.

So, how can you tell if you have normal anxiety or have a disorder? Mental health professionals often refer to the *Diagnostic and Statistical Manual of Mental Disorders (DSM-5)* for the guidelines for making a diagnosis. An anxiety disorder is diagnosed when:

- The anxiety one experiences are excessive: being afraid of snakes may be normal but being petrified of worms would be considered extreme.
- The anxiety is constant and can last for weeks or months at a time: there are different time frames for each type of disorder. For example, when panic disorder symptoms last for a month or more, it can be diagnosed as an anxiety disorder. However, for generalized anxiety disorder, the symptoms must be present for a minimum of six months.
- The anxiety itself causes more anxiety: when a person becomes really upset by the mere fact that they are experiencing anxiety.
- The anxiety interferes with a person's normal activities: when you can't walk outside of your home, go into a public place, or can't work on a job because of the heightened level of anxiety.

There are several different types of anxieties that could be considered an anxiety disorder. They are very different from each other, so before treatment can be started, one must understand exactly what type of disorder they have.

Phobias: Phobias are powerful and irrational fears of a particular object or situation. Common phobias could be a fear of anything from snakes to something that is part of the natural environment. Most common forms of phobias might be an extreme fear of storms, flying, elevators, spiders, and even people. In many cases, these start with a traumatic experience, but not always. Sometimes, the actual cause of a phobia is never discovered.

Social Anxiety Disorder (SAD): These are fears of social situations. In these types of cases, the fear is often confined to the fear of embarrassment. SAD is different from other phobias because it often involves the mind "guessing" about what is going to happen or what someone else might be thinking. With other phobias, we may know that the thing we're imagining can actually happen. We know about dog and snake bites; there is plenty evidence of the consequences of such events, but social phobias are more likely related to what one might be thinking rather than as a result of what they believe.

Panic Disorders: Panic disorders usually come about without warning. Many often mistake a panic attack for a disorder, but panic attacks that might be experienced are usually the symptom of the fear or phobia of a certain situation.

The attacks come on suddenly like a loud alarm going off in the body. The sympathetic nervous system instantly triggers a "fight-or-flight" response that is very physical. It releases a huge dose of adrenaline into the system to help prepare the body for danger. As a result, the person will experience:

- Rapid heartbeat
- Faster and deeper breathing
- Dizziness
- Profuse sweating
- Digestive problems
- Tense muscles

A person may experience some of these symptoms or all, but the concept here is that the symptoms are not just a little change but are quite extreme.

Agoraphobia: Interestingly enough, agoraphobia is not a very specific phobia but is the fear of being in places where you feel it would be bad to have a panic attack. This causes the person to avoid public areas such as movie theaters, shopping centers, public transportation, etc. If they go anywhere at all, it is usually in the company of another person they feel is safe and would be able to help them if something were to happen. In extreme cases, the patient is reluctant to leave the house at all and may squirrel away inside for years at a time.

General Anxiety Disorder (GAD): This disorder presents itself as a persistent and pervasive sense of worry. It is not the normal concerns of everyday life that most people have but is so intrusive that it interrupts sleep, keeps the individual from concentrating which leaves them to feel exhausted all the time. Unlike other anxiety disorders, GAD is also evidenced by anxiety and worries that are spread out over a number of different areas. It is not specific to a single type of fear, thus the name of General Anxiety Disorder. The individual's life is plagued by a never-ending worry about "what ifs" to the point that they can no longer function normally.

People who suffer from panic attacks, phobias, obsessive thoughts, and a never-ending stream of worries about everything will gain the most from CBT. This type of therapy, unlike medications, treats much more than just the symptoms that you may have. It can help to reveal the underlying causes of those incessant worries and fears. As a result, patients learn to relax and see each situation in a completely fresh and less intimidating way. They become better at coping and learn how to think through all of their problems.

There are many different types of anxiety disorders, so each session will be tailored to the specific problem of each patient. For example, for those who may be struggling with obsessive-compulsive disorder (OCD), their treatment will differ greatly from someone who is struggling with an anxiety attack.

The therapist will work with them to first identify the negative thought and then teach them through guided sessions on how to challenge those thoughts. For example:

Negative thought: What if I have a panic attack on the subway? I'll pass out!

Distortion: Believing that only the worst can happen.

Challenge: Have you ever passed out on the subway before? It's unlikely that you will pass out on the subway.

Negative thought: If I pass out, terrible things will happen.

Distortion: Expectations clearly out of proportion with reality.

Challenge: If I do pass out, it'll only be for a few seconds. That's not so bad.

Negative thought: People will think I'm crazy.

Distortion: Drawing conclusions you know nothing about.

Challenge: People are more likely to show concern and help.

In the beginning, these thought challenges will be guided with the therapist, but in time, the patient will learn to do these themselves. For milder cases, an individual can work these out for themselves with the use of a CBT workbook. Negative thinking doesn't just happen all on its own but is an accumulation of a lifetime of negative influences. While it sounds simple here, it can be quite difficult to remold one's thinking into something that is more positive. Those suffering from anxiety and depression disorders will:

- Learn to identify anxiety and how it feels in the body
- Learn skills to help them to cope and relax to counteract the anxiety
- Learn to confront their fears (real or not)

Of all the psychological disorders you can find, anxiety is by far the most common.

- 18% of anxiety disorders are phobias
- 13% are social anxiety disorders
- 9% are general anxiety disorders
- 7% are panic disorders
- 4% are agoraphobia

Depressive Disorders

Depressive disorders come in a different form. Many may start with some type of injury that renders them unable to function for a time. This triggers a train of losses or disappointments of many of the things the person may use to enjoy. The loss of these once fulfilling activities starts him on a downward spiral where he begins to believe that he doesn't deserve them or that he's done something that has triggered the loss.

A depressive disorder can make it difficult to function in any capacity. They may feel like everything they do is ten times harder than it used to be. It could feel like trying to pull themselves out of a quicksand and they may feel that they are so pathetic or worthless that it is not worth putting up the effort.

Most people only know depression as a feeling of sadness, but its symptoms can vary widely depending on the type of depression they are experiencing. It can present itself in many forms. In many cases, the patient has no idea that he or she

144

is dealing with depression, because often, the symptoms do not present themselves as they would expect.

Major Depressive Disorder: Another term for someone who is "clinically depressed" is a major depressive disorder. This can be described as a person who feels low for the better part of the day. However, while this is a very common symptom, it is not necessary for them to feel an overwhelming sense of sadness to be considered depressed. It could be evident in their lack of interest in any activities, many of which they may have used to enjoy.

At the same time, they may sleep excessively, eat more than usual (whether they are hungry or not), or stop eating altogether. They feel exhausted and have a hard time concentrating on what they need to do or even making decisions.

While we all have a tendency to feel bad about ourselves at one time or another, those who are clinically depressed feel so bad about themselves that they believe they are completely worthless and are at a very high risk of suicidal tendencies, so they need to be watched carefully.

According to DSM-5, there are nine different symptoms of depression; five are needed to be observed in order to be diagnosed as clinically depressed. Because of this, the condition of depression may look very different from one person to the next.

Persistent Depressive Disorder: There are ebbs and flows of a major depressive disorder, where the individual may feel up and good at times but at other times, they may struggle to even get out of bed. With a persistent depressive disorder, however, the symptoms may seem to be more chronic. To be diagnosed with a persistent depressive disorder, they have to experience symptoms consistently for a minimum of two years before they are diagnosed. In addition, they need to display at least two more symptoms listed in the DSM-5.

With a PDD, the symptoms can be milder, but its negative effects can be extreme. While the symptoms may not appear to be as severe as an MDD, one can never assume that its effects are not as bad. At times, the symptoms can be even more destructive because of their chronic nature, as the individual never gets any sort of relief from the pervasive symptoms.

Premenstrual Dysphoric Disorder: This type of depression usually appears just before and for several days into a woman's menstrual period. It is important to understand that this is not the same thing as PMS (premenstrual syndrome). The condition is much more extreme with women displaying volatile mood swings and irritability. In addition to feeling anxiety, they can often show physical symptoms as well including breast tenderness and bloating. The symptoms should appear before or during most of her menstrual cycles for as much as a year before being accurately diagnosed.

Getting diagnosed with an anxiety or a mood disorder is not always easy. In fact, the process can be quite complex. Each form of depression has to have a number of different labels that identify exactly which type of depression the person may be dealing with and its nature. In addition to the main symptoms listed above, there may be seasonal depression, postpartum, a form of melancholy, single, and recurrent episodes. Whatever the case, there is a good chance that applying CBT techniques can help to manage all of these symptoms. One of the first things an individual needs to do is to get an official diagnosis. Once the diagnosis is completed, the next step is to sit down and work out how it is affecting you in order to determine the goals you want to work towards and a time frame in which to complete them in.

How CBT Helps With Substance Abuse

While CBT is most often used for anxiety and depressive disorders, there are many more mental health issues that it can also help with. It has been highly effective in preventing the relapse of problem drinking and drug addictions. These are common behavioral patterns that can be readjusted by redirecting the thought processes that trigger the abuse of many substances.

A key element of CBT is teaching the patient to anticipate situations and give them practical strategies to help them to cope effectively when these conditions arise. These strategies could include things like analyzing consequences before a decision is made to use the substance, self-monitoring themselves so they can identify cravings at the onset, and avoid situations where they might be at a higher risk of using.

By learning to develop strategies that will help them to better deal with cravings and those situations where they will find themselves more vulnerable, they can reduce and eventually eliminate their use of these substances

With the treatment for substance abuse, the objective of CBT is to:

- Help the individual to identify those situations where they are more likely to use alcohol or drugs
- Help them to develop strategies to avoid such situations
- And to identify common problems and triggers, which could cause them to abuse substances

This is done through two major components: function analysis and skills training.

With functional analysis, the therapist and the individual works to identify certain thoughts, feelings, and environments that historically have led to substance abuse. From this, they are able to determine the level of risk the patient is likely to face, or under what situations could expose them to a potential relapse.

CBT also will give them special insight into what started them on the path to substance abuse in the first place. Then they will give them coping strategies, so they are equipped to handle similar situations in the future.

With skills training, the individual will learn better coping skills. They will work on unlearning those old habits that took them in the wrong direction and replacing them with healthier habits that will be of benefit to them. In other words, they will be educated about how to change their thinking so that they are better able to deal with the varying situations that will trigger more episodes in the future.

To date, more than 24 different trials have been conducted with substance abusers of all sorts including those who are addicted to alcohol, cocaine, marijuana, opiates, and tobacco. In each of these studies, CBT has proven to be one of the most effective forms of treatment in helping to restructure their recovery. However, it is not the catchall answer for everyone. Because each person is different in the nature of their problems, everyone will respond to this type of treatment in a different way. Still, the results speak for themselves and if you or someone you care about is struggling with some form of substance abuse, there is a good chance that they will learn something and gain some benefit from incorporating CBT into their lives.

Chapter 2: How CBT Can Help With…

We live in unpredictable times and every one of us may be expected to address a number of issues at any given time. It can be a pretty stressful life for most of us. However, if someone is dealing with intrusive thoughts on top of the problems they face, it can become a complex maze that they may struggle desperately to get out of.

Dealing with any problem is not really the issue for these people. When a situation arises, the difficulty occurs with the manner in which he or she may address it. If their solution is based on distorted thinking, it can create a myriad of new problems in addition to creating a snowball effect. People who are plagued with unrealistic and intrusive thoughts are usually more reactionary rather than taking a proactive approach.

CBT's goal-oriented approach encourages a hands-on and more practical direction which teaches the patient that there is a means to an end. They do this by making a comparison between where the individual is at the start of the problem and then working out the best path to take to achieve the set goal. The ultimate goal is to change the thought pattern, which in turn, will change how they feel, and by extension, their behavior. In this way, CBT has been used to treat a wide variety of problems that range from sleep disorders to relationship issues.

On the surface, the logic of CBT is very simple: change one's negative thinking to positive thinking. However, this is not always easy. It requires that the person first learn to identify the negative thought processes they have. This requires them to take a hard look at themselves and give an honest appraisal of how they really think.

This may involve applying a little mindfulness and seeing their thoughts as a neutral person. When they see that their views are overly negative or overly positive. They will be compelled to learn to adopt a more balanced view of themselves, those around them, and their environment; viewing everything as a neutral person. This kind of adjustment takes time, as they may not fully realize just how far their thinking has strayed from the normal way of things.

Patients need to learn how to identify when their thoughts are triggering negative emotions and when to stop them before this happens. Then, they need to examine those thoughts honestly to determine if they are truly giving a fair and honest appraisal of the situation; how realistic they are and how damaging those thoughts are to them.

This helps them to avoid falling into thinking traps (negative ways of viewing things) so they don't fall into the problem situation in the first place. These mental traps could become major landmines that could quickly throw them into a world of trouble. These thinking traps are often negative words they would never say to others, but they say it to themselves.

Consider if you don't like people talking down to you, then why would you do the same thing to yourself? It is possible to hurt your own feelings and damage your self-esteem. One of the first traps they are taught to avoid is those that you do without realizing it. Through CBT, you learn to identify these habits, stop them, and then change that point of view.

Problem-Solving With Depression or Anxiety

Problem-solving therapy empowers people, so they are better equipped to change the circumstances of their lives. They learn to work through challenges and take a proactive approach to their problems. Through this type of program, patients learn how to manage these issues through several core components:

Addressing the Problem: There are many approaches that people can take when they deal with a problem. Some will naturally be more submissive in the decision-making phase, others will apply avoidance techniques, and others will be more aggressive. Whatever strategy one takes, the treatment will focus on the developing thoughts and attitudes one applies to solve their particular problems. It will work to identify certain weaknesses and address those with cognitive steps and techniques.

Defining the Problem: The next step is to define exactly what the problem is so they have a clear understanding of what they are dealing with. For example, a client may see that they are constantly under stress while at work. The first conclusion might be that they are dealing with anxiety. However, other factors may be at the root of the anxiety. They may not be assertive enough on the job and as a result, are allowing people to overburden them with additional work. They may not be setting boundaries, so people do not know their limits, and this is adding to their stress level.

Developing Strategies to Help Them Cope: Together, they work with the therapist to outline very specific steps that will help them to change their behavior and provide a number of possible solutions to the problem. By taking into consideration a wide variety of possibilities that will work, they may feel more empowered and actually begin to believe that they can work it out.

Execution: Finally, when they have broken down their goals into smaller easy-to-achieve steps, they are better capable of taking the necessary action to solve the problem. As they progress through the different steps, they will gain confidence and are more likely to follow the plan and successfully solve their problems.

There have been many studies that have definitively shown that this type of therapy can be a very useful form of therapy on its own. However, it can be even more effective when it is included in a full CBT treatment plan, yielding even better results.

CBT with Sleep Disorders

Often, people who struggle with sleep disorders have an extremely difficult time dealing with life in general. With a lack of sleep, they will naturally suffer from low energy, and when their energy is low, they are likely to also have poor nutrition. Poor nutrition contributes to brain fogginess, and in the end, they are caught up in a vicious cycle that is difficult for them to break free from. CBT can help them to get to the root cause of their sleep disorder and correct the wayward thoughts that are interrupting their ability to sleep.

Insomnia, a common sleep disorder that affects many people, has been treated very effectively through CBT. The condition makes it hard to fall asleep and even more difficult to stay asleep once you do.

CBT-1, the form of therapy used for sleep disorders, is a structured program that helps you to replace those intrusive thoughts with the kind of habits that will be more conducive to getting good sleep. The right treatment used for your sleep disorder will depend on a variety of factors.

Stimulus Control Therapy: This form of therapy focuses on removing the factors that may be contributing to your inability to sleep. These could include setting up routines that will support a better bedtime routine, one that is more conducive to sleep. It may involve setting up a consistent time to go to bed and wake up, avoiding naps, and restricting the use of the bed for anything other than sleeping and sex. No eating, watching TV or talking on the phone while in bed.

Sleep Restriction: This treatment would prevent you from being in bed for too long a time without sleeping. If you're in bed for more than 20 minutes without sleeping, it can add to your sleep deprivation. With sleep restriction, the amount of time you spend in the bed is shortened to only when you can sleep. Once you have developed a healthy sleep period, this time can be extended until you reach a point where you can sleep through the night.

Sleep Hygiene: This will get rid of those negative habits that interrupt sleep. Smoking, too much caffeine late in the day, consuming too much alcohol, or lack of exercise can all be part of the problem. CBT therapy can help you to reduce or eliminate those habits so that you can more easily relax before bedtime.

Sleep Environment Improvement: This treatment focuses on habits that create a positive sleep environment. Strategies to keep the room dark, quiet, and at the right temperature can be very effective in teaching a patient to relax.

Passive Awakeness: This focuses on avoiding any attempt to fall asleep. Interestingly enough, worrying about not being able to sleep can contribute to one's inability to sleep. Learning how to not worry about it allows the body to relax so you can drift off to sleep more easily.

Biofeedback: Once a person is aware of how his biological functions are operating, they can learn how to manipulate them. Many of these factors can interrupt one's sleep. A person's heart rate, tension in their muscles, or body temperature can all interfere with their regular sleep patterns. Learning how to mentally adjust these and other biological elements can put your body into a more comfortable state where sleep will come easily.

Whether your sleep disorder is mild or extreme, using CBT-1 can help all sorts of problems. Even if the cause of the problem is physical, as in cases of chronic pain, or mental, as in cases of anxiety and depression, the problems tend to go away once the right kind of therapy is undertaken, all without negative side effects. It will require consistent practice and applications, but the longer you stick with it, the better the end results will be.

Chapter 3: Common Causes of Mood Disorders

When you first start Cognitive Behavioral Therapy, one of the first things you will have to do is to identify the root cause of your dysfunction. In nearly every case, the problem lies in your automatic thoughts. These are at the heart of the theory behind this type of treatment.

Automatic thoughts are known to pop into your mind without any effort. They are the brain's means of processing all of the information it is receiving from the environment. These thoughts do not represent any type of fact about the situation that it is processing, which is why they can cause so much damage. The type of automatic thoughts that appear immediately after dealing with a specific situation can be referred to as your "instinctive" response. They appear so quickly that there is literally no time to reason on the situation or apply logic, so relying on them to make decisions is often the reason why a person would display dysfunctional behavior.

In your first session with the therapist, you will learn to recognize your dysfunctional thoughts. Likely, you will backtrack from a specific experience in order to identify the actual thought that triggered your negative emotion. You should pay close attention to any thoughts that cause you to have a reflex change in mood in response to it. These are the dangerous thoughts that are connected to what you truly believe about something.

A good example of this may be how you react when you watch someone speaking in public. Your knee-jerk reaction to what is said is a reflection of what you truly believe about that situation. If there is a great deal of approval from the audience but you don't like it, your mind won't take the time to contemplate his words. If you are applying your feelings to yourself, your thoughts might reflect a general negativity about yourself. "People will never respond to me like that," or "I wish

I was as happy as he is." These personal negative reflections are labeled as "dysfunctional automatic thoughts." These beliefs will trigger equally negative feelings that are, in turn, triggering certain behaviors you want to change.

To address these thoughts through CBT, you will first have to figure out if your negative thought patterns are caused by a physical imbalance in your system. There are several things that could tell if you are physically out of balance.

Chemical Imbalances

There is quite a bit of dispute about whether chemical imbalances are a real cause of mental disorders or not. It was once believed that chemical imbalances are the result of too much of some chemicals or too little being produced in the brain. These chemicals, called neurotransmitters, are used to aid in the communication between the neurons of the brain. You may have heard of many of them: dopamine, serotonin, and norepinephrine are just a few. It was generally understood in the world of psychiatry that mental disorders like depression and anxiety are usually the result of these chemicals being out of balance in the brain.

These types of disorders can be extremely complex, and finding a definitive answer to your problem is not always easy. However, a good way to assess whether or not you're dealing with these types of imbalances is by looking at the symptoms.

- Feeling sad, worthless, or empty
- Tendency to overeat
- Loss of appetite
- Inability to sleep
- Sleeping too much
- Feeling restless
- Irritable

- A constant feeling of dread
- Listless
- Not wanting to associate with others
- Lacking empathy
- Feeling numb all over
- Extreme mood swings
- Inability to concentrate
- Suicidal thoughts
- Thoughts of hurting others
- Inability to perform normal everyday activities
- Hearing voices that are not there
- Substance abuse

While we don't know the exact cause of these imbalances, many researchers believe that it could be a combination of genetics, our environment, and social influences on our lives. It is even unclear how these are able to affect us and create mental disorders. What we do know is that even if you do have a chemical imbalance, it is not the end of the situation. By applying the techniques of CBT, it is possible to change to more positive behaviors, which can, in time, correct them.

Dopamine: The brain uses dopamine to control both your movements and your emotional responses. When it is balanced properly, it is an essential component for physical and mental wellbeing. It also helps facilitate important brain functions like your mood, your ability to sleep, how you learn, concentration, motor control, and even the ability to remember things. If you are low in dopamine, you are likely to feel:

- Muscle cramps
- Tremors

- Aches and pains
- Stiffness in the muscles
- Have difficulty keep your balance
- Constipation
- Trouble eating or swallowing
- An unexplainable weight loss or weight gain
- Gastroesophageal reflux disease
- Trouble sleeping
- Low energy
- Poor concentration
- Excessive fatigue
- Unmotivated
- Extreme sadness or hopelessness
- Poor self-esteem
- Anxiety
- Suicidal thoughts
- Low libido
- A lack of self-awareness

A dopamine deficiency may be linked to a number of mental health disorders. It may not be the direct cause, but it can certainly contribute to the severity of the problem.

Serotonin: While your body mostly uses serotonin in the digestive system, it can have an effect on every part of your body including your emotions. It can also be found in the blood platelets and in various parts of the central nervous system. It is made from tryptophan, an amino acid found in common foods like nuts, cheese, and red meat. When you have a deficiency of serotonin, it can trigger anxiety or depressive mood disorders.

Because it can be found throughout the body, it can have a major impact on everything from your emotions to your motor skills. It is the body's natural way of keeping the mood stable. It also helps with eating, digesting foods, and allowing us to relax enough so we can sleep. When you have a good balance of serotonin, your body can:

- Fight off depression
- Control levels of anxiety
- Heal wounds better
- Maintain good bone health

You will also find that you are:

- Happier
- Emotionally stable
- Calmer
- Less anxious
- Able to concentrate better

If your serotonin levels are too high, it could be a sign of carcinoid syndrome, a condition that causes tumors in the small intestine, bronchial tubes, appendix, or the colon. Your doctor could determine your serotonin levels through a simple blood test. Symptoms of a serotonin deficiency are:

- Poor memory
- Signs of aggression
- Low or depressed mood
- Anxiety
- Cravings for sweet or starchy foods
- Insomnia
- Low self-esteem

You are equally at risk of major health problems if your serotonin levels are too high or too low, so it is very important to keep a good balance to protect not just your physical health but your mental health as well.

Other Imbalances: There are other chemicals in the brain that can have an effect on your moods and emotions. However, as we now understand how the brain works, it is important to realize that there is still an ongoing debate as to what extent these imbalances actually cause or affect the moods and emotions.

It should be a foregone conclusion that no person is born with these anxiety disorders. Whether the imbalances are a result of one's genetic make-up or are from the environment, it is clear that there is only one way that we know of to fix it. We have already learned that habits and behaviors are developed by using the neural pathways in the brain to send signals back and forth. Since these chemicals are responsible for facilitating that communication, it only stands to reason that the best way to treat imbalances is to strengthen those connections.

Because it focuses on those automatic thoughts, even if there is a chemical imbalance, it can be reversed by regular practice of the routine steps and strategies a patient will learn while working through the steps of CBT.

Chapter 4: Understanding Your Moods and the Way You Think

Understanding your mood and the way you think is not easy. As you analyze a particular situation where you have been feeling those negative emotions, you have to start with a serious self-analysis. Your goal is to figure out exactly what kind of thoughts and feelings you have lying just underneath the surface. You can do this by asking yourself some very pointed questions:

- What was I doing when I began to feel that way?
- Where was I?
- Is this the only place where I feel like this?
- What was my behavior like before and after this episode?
- What hidden beliefs do I have that are showing right now?
- What causes me to intensify those feelings?
- Who was I with?
- Am I the same with everyone or just certain people?

An honest answer to these types of questions can be very revealing. For example, a person may start to feel depressed when he is alone and away from other people. These types of questions help you to get to exactly why you have experienced those sudden mood changes. If you're a person that suddenly feels awkward and ashamed when you're in the gym, you may be harboring hidden beliefs in relation to your body image. If you start to feel negative emotions while out in public, it could mean that you have serious concerns about your abilities to perform in front of strangers.

After doing this type of exercise, most people are surprised when they learn so much about themselves this way. It can be alarming to discover that their automatic thoughts, which are often just fleeting in the mind, can have such power, triggering emotions unexpectedly as if they just came on without warning. Usually, these thoughts reveal a very specific issue and once you know what it is, you can now direct your energy to that particular thought process.

How to Diagnose Your Negative Thought Patterns

As you get started working your way through this stage of therapy, you must realize that no two people will have the exact same disorder. While they may have been diagnosed with the same label, your personal experience will be very different from someone else, because you bring to it your own personal body of experiences.

Even finding the answers to questions like the ones listed above are not easy to do. You may have to get a frank viewpoint from someone close to you and whom you can trust to get the ball rolling. Some complete the entire first session without learning what is at the heart of their problem. However, they will have learned how to start trying to think differently about their experiences.

This is not to be surprising. Most of us have gotten pretty good at hiding some of those negatives that permeate our lives every day and have done so for years. It's not likely that everything is going to come out in the first wash. Still, if you persist in this type of self-analysis, there is a very good chance that you will be able to identify many of the tricks and tactics you have created to cover up your true feelings about certain things.

As you go through this process, don't be afraid to look at every aspect of your life and not just in the obvious areas. It is quite often that the real trigger has little or no direct connection to where your thinking went awry. For example, you may be having a communication problem with your spouse. He or she may think you are distant, uncommunicative, or just has lost interest in the relationship. However, if you're dealing with a hidden anxiety or depression that started many years prior, it may still be affecting you and causing you to separate from your partner.

Imagine it this way. You are a child and you have a close and dear friend who died of a sudden illness. Your relationship was strong, and you were always very happy when with that person. However, their death suddenly left a huge void in your life. On the surface, you were able to eventually get over it and move on, but that pain was never clearly addressed. Now, in a relationship, you are afraid to commit that way to another person.

This kind of hidden pain could be what is causing those automatic thoughts that are firing in your brain.

- I can't commit to another person, they will leave me.
- I can't go through losing someone again in my life.
- It's not worth it. Everybody is going to die anyway.

A past loss may have been the real reason you don't trust or are afraid to communicate with your spouse. People die, friends move away, jobs are lost, and a myriad of other conditions could be behind the reason for your automatic thoughts. If you were a child when it happened, it is quite possible your grief was either not recognized or considered unimportant in a world where everyone else is in grief too. However, being able to learn the hidden secrets that are triggering those automatic thoughts can give you great insight on where they come from and why they are resurfacing. As a result, you have a basis for addressing the issue now and correcting those thoughts from a more realistic position.

Now, this may seem strange in light of what we said earlier; that a CBT therapist does not reach back into our past to find the root cause of a problem. This is true, however, as you begin to recognize these automatic thoughts, it is only a small step to making the connection between your past and the present.

Once you are able to identify those thoughts, there are several ways you can deal with them.

- If you feel the thought is indicative of a larger issue, you can choose to put all your energies into correcting that thought.
- If you feel that there is another problem that better identifies the issue, you can choose to focus on the two thoughts together.
- If you discover that there are other issues that are beginning to surface, you can put the initial thought aside and focus on the bigger and most important issues first.

After you have uncovered these hidden thoughts, the next step is to analyze each thought and rate them as to how important they are. If one thought seems to produce intense feelings in one way or another, it is likely the one that has the biggest impact.

Sometimes, it can be difficult to separate the different thoughts in your mind. In that case, it is helpful to keep a notepad nearby and write down the thoughts as they appear. As you write down each thought, make sure to also take note of what was happening when it occurred and the feelings it evoked. If you do this over a period of time (perhaps a week), you'll begin to notice a definite pattern emerge.

There are several different categories of automatic thoughts, and by journaling them as they happen, the patterns that emerge will help you to classify the type of thoughts you're having. Below is a list of some of the most common beliefs that many people develop that can trigger negative emotions.

- All or nothing: A person who believes everything is either black or white with no middle ground or gray area.
- Catastrophizing: A belief that every situation will produce the worst results.

- Discounting Positives: The belief that all positive experiences are false.

- Emotional Reasoning: Allowing one's negative feelings about a situation to be the deciding voice in their head.

- Jumping to Conclusions: Automatically concluding negative results for a situation with any evidence to back up assumptions.

- Labeling: The act of giving negative labels to ourselves or to other people. Calling yourself a loser or a failure rather than making the effort to change the quality you don't like.

- Magnification/Minimization: Putting a lot of emphasis on anything bad and downgrading anything good. Really stressing out about a mistake but not willing to accept compliments or acknowledge achievements.

- Negative Bias: Seeing only the bad in any situation and dwelling on the negative, despite the fact that there are many positives.

- Overgeneralizations: Using a single negative experience to represent every other similar event.

- Personalization: Believing that negative comments or actions from others are about you or believing that you are the cause of a bad event even when you had no connection with it.

- Should/Must statements: Having expectations based on what you believe should be done. These often stem from distorted perceptions of what others may believe about you and are likely not in the realm of reality. This could cause you to feel guilty for not meeting these abstract standards or often excessively high expectations.

Likely, as you read through this list, some of these dysfunctional automatic thoughts popped out at you. All of us have them from time to time, but if you think they are interfering with the progression in your life, then these should be the ones that you should focus your CBT exercises on.

Intrusive Thoughts

In our minds, we have many thoughts throughout the course of a single day. It is estimated that each of us has between 50-70,000 thoughts in a single 24-hour period. Most of them, we are able to quickly dismiss as insignificant and unimportant. But there are those disturbing thoughts that seem to get stuck in our brain and no matter what we do; we can't seem to get rid of them. They make us feel sad, frightened, and sometimes, even sick and can create a great deal of turmoil in our emotions.

The fact that they are so intrusive and they seem to camp out in our head can cause us even more distress; some to the point where they interfere with our regular routines and activities causing us to feel ashamed, guilty, or afraid. Anyone suffering from an anxiety disorder like OCD or PTSD can quickly relate to the kind of damage an intrusive thought like these can do.

These thoughts are always unpleasant and can even make you feel repulsed. They can include acts of violence, inappropriate sexual acts, or extreme criminal behavior. Those in relation to anxiety could be an excessive worry about future events or threats. Strategies learned through CBT can help to reduce their frequency and even help to lessen the extremes that they may take. Addressing these feelings would be a good way to start getting rid of them.

Examples of Some Intrusive Thoughts

- Unwanted sexual fantasies involving a child, animal, or another person close to you
- Unwanted sexual thoughts involving someone you work with but are not really attracted to.
- Imagining yourself committing a violent criminal act
- Fear that you will say the wrong thing in public

- Doubts about your religion or thoughts of doing something forbidden
- Doubts about your inability to do well on an exam you know you have prepared for
- Recurring thoughts about getting a rare disease
- Fear of death
- Repeated memories about something humiliating that happened in your childhood
- Repeated memories about a violent experience you had in the past

It is important to know at this point, that having intrusive thoughts is not indicative of a disorder. Everyone has them at one point or another. According to the *Journal of Obsessive-Compulsive Disorders*, 94% of people in the world have intrusive thoughts. It is one of the most common mental activities that we all have. What is different in those who have anxiety or depressive disorders is our reaction to those thoughts.

When you are healthy and your mental state is balanced, you are able to dismiss those thoughts and they won't upset you. When you struggle with those thoughts, it is because you have already associated a great deal of importance to them, which is an indication that you have an internal belief that they are true and accurate. In such cases, your mind starts to create a full narrative about those thoughts and conjure up its own implications about what kind of behavior you should display or what your future actions should be.

To counteract these thoughts, one of the first things you need to do is analyze them, so you can convince yourself that they are NOT true. This is especially important when you are dealing with some of the above thoughts that may be violent or otherwise inappropriate. It does not mean that you really want to do those things. If you continue to accept these things as true, then it can saddle you with an immeasurable sense of guilt and shame, which could cause you even more problems.

If you're struggling with these types of intrusive thoughts, then take some of the following steps to apply some CBT-based strategies to combat them.

Identifying Your Triggers for Anxiety and Stress

It is one thing to know what your problem is and another thing entirely to identify what is triggering the symptoms you're experiencing. Finding these triggers can be quite complicated as it is most likely due to a combination of factors including environmental, physical, and genetics. Even so, there are some events or personal experiences that may trigger certain forms of anxiety or, at the very least, make them much worse.

So, whether you're dealing with symptoms of anxiety, depression, or stress as a result of a genetic factor that you have no control over, the condition can actually deepen as a result of certain events or experiences you are having in your day-to-day life. These events, emotions, and experiences are called triggers.

These triggers can vary from one person to the next. However, in most cases, you're likely responding to several triggers at one time. It may seem, on the surface, that your reaction to a given situation comes completely out of nowhere, but in most cases, there is always something there, just underneath the surface. So, while it may be uncomfortable to do, it is important to root out your personal triggers, so you can take proactive steps in managing them. Below are some of the most common triggers that many people have.

Health Issues: Often, your own health may be playing a part in increasing your anxiety or depression. Diseases such as cancer or another type of chronic illness can trigger anxiety or even make it worse. Just getting a diagnosis of a disease like cancer can immediately evoke powerfully negative emotions that can be very difficult to combat.

To counteract this kind of trigger, you need to take a proactive approach by working together with your doctor and even discussing it with a therapist as they can give you strategies to help you manage your emotions as you go through your treatment.

Medications: The intrusive thoughts and negative emotions may be the result of the medication you're taking. While there is always a risk with certain prescription drugs of generating negative thoughts, even over-the-counter medications have been known to trigger anxiety and/or depression. This is due to the active ingredients that are working on your system. If you are able to dismiss these thoughts as a result of the medication, then great, but many people do not realize that the feelings they generate can trigger a number of side effects that could increase your level of anxiety.

Common medications that have been known to trigger anxiety/depression:

- birth control pills
- cold/flu medications to treat a cough and congestion
- weight loss medications

While for most people the symptoms will be non-existent or minimal, for those who have anxiety and depression disorders, these could pose a real problem. If after taking any medication, you find the intrusive thoughts are increasing or are causing negative emotions, speak with your doctor and get him/her to help you find an acceptable alternative.

Caffeine: Believe it or not, many people are addicted to caffeine, not realizing that it can be a very strong trigger for anxiety. Research has shown that people who are already susceptible to panic disorders or social anxiety disorders will be even more sensitive to the negative effects of caffeine.

To combat this, one of the best things you can do is to reduce or eliminate the amount of caffeine you consume and substitute it with other options for the stimulation you need.

Your Diet: Believe it or not, your diet can be a major contributing factor to your mental stability. Skipping meals, especially, can have a negative impact on your mental state. When you miss a meal, it causes your blood sugar levels to drop, which can trigger anxiety along with a host of other symptoms including that jittery feeling, nervousness, or agitation.

The best way to counteract this problem is to eat regularly and make sure that you have a diet that is balanced so that you get an adequate amount of nutrients in your system. The old rule that you must eat 3-5 meals a day is no longer encouraged. However, you need to make sure that your diet consists of enough nutrients to sustain you on a daily basis to prevent a drop in blood sugar.

Negativity: Nothing happens in our body unless it first happens in our mind, including anxiety. Your brain is the control center for your entire body so when you have anxiety, your self-talk can have a major impact on how you function. If you tend to be negative in your conversation or you are known for using a lot of negativity in reference to yourself, it can create a perpetual negative outlook on everything you do. Learn to use more positive expressions in your conversation and your feelings will soon follow. If you find this difficult, consider working with a therapist for a while until you learn to change your automatic conversation to a more positive and up-building form of self-talk.

Financial Problems: Debt can be a painful burden to undergo. Constant worry about not having enough or finding ways to save money can trigger a great deal of anxiety. While you may not be able to change your circumstances immediately, learning to manage these types of triggers can help to ease a lot of your intrusive thoughts. Working with a therapist can help guide you to a process that could help to get your mind to relax more.

Public Situations: Often, public events that include a lot of strangers can make one feel uncomfortable. The pressure of having to interact feels like walking through unfamiliar territory and can trigger many anxious feelings.

Worries about such occasions can be reduced by asking a trusted friend to accompany you so you won't feel like you're on your own. If your anxiety about these things is particularly intense, consider learning some coping mechanisms from a professional therapist so you are better equipped to managing them.

Conflict: Conflict in any form can be very stressful. Whether it is a relationship problem or a disagreement at work, these can trigger some of the worse anxiety you can deal with. If this is becoming a particularly stressful area for you, consider learning some conflict resolution strategies to learn better ways to control your feelings when conflicts arise.

Stress: We all face stress on a daily basis, but some of us get a bigger dose of it than others. Daily stress, when it is intense and constant, can trigger extreme anxiety symptoms along with other health problems. When under stress, you are likely picking up other habits that will contribute to your anxiety levels. Habits like over drinking, skipping meals, or insomnia will only intensify the anxiety.

Learning to first identify these habits and a few coping mechanisms will help you to handle them better so that they aren't allowed to overwhelm you.

Public Events/Performances: Situations that require you to speak or perform in public can be extremely stressful. Whether it is speaking up at a business meeting or competing at a special event, the stress can trigger all sorts of negative emotions and behaviors.

Try working along with a trusted friend or relative with some positive reinforcement to help you prepare and feel more comfortable beforehand. Regular practice with people you trust and even having them along with you for support can help you to feel more confident and relaxed.

Your Own Personal Triggers: It may be that you have triggers that are unique to you. These may not be so easy to identify. They could be something as simple as a smell that triggers something in your mind, the sounds of a song, the resemblance of a place or any number of things that can bring back a memory of a past traumatic event. This is common with people who suffer from PTSD. The triggers could be any number of things in their environment.

If you can identify these triggers, you can then take the next step to address them. Since these personal triggers are not likely to be those experienced by others, you will have to do a little bit of soul searching to uncover them. To help you find them, try these tips:

- Start keeping a journal where you take note of when your anxiety or depression is heightened. Record your thoughts and your feelings that occur at the same time. For example, answer the 5 W's (who, what, when, where, and why). After a while, you'll be able to see a certain pattern begin to emerge that will give you clues to your triggers.

- Be honest with yourself. Negative self-talk stems from a poor assessment of your true values and qualities. As long as you stay within that negative mode, it will be difficult to uncover the triggers to your anxiety and depression. Don't just accept the first thing that comes in your head. Be patient and be willing to look a little deeper into your life (past and present) to identify how they are making you feel.

- If the above two tips don't work, consider spending some time with a therapist. Even with all the effort you put out, some triggers have been so well-hidden that no matter what you do, it will be hard to pull out. Working with a professional can make it easier and take a lot of the pressure off of you.

Once you know and have identified your triggers, you have accomplished the first step in Cognitive Behavioral Therapy. Now, you can make a list of the problems you're facing and choose the ones you'd like to address and you're ready to move on to the next step in CBT.

Chapter 5: How it Treats Mood Disorders

During your first week of CBT, after you've identified the major problems you want to address, you'll have to go into setting goals for yourself. You know the type of anxiety and depression you're experiencing. Now, you need to work on a system for addressing these issues.

Practical Applications of CBT

Since no two forms of anxiety or depressive disorders are the same, there is no single way to deal with the challenges that each individual may face. Even those with the same diagnosis will have a different approach to their treatment. This means that before setting your goals, you need to have a pretty clear idea of what your specific problem is and what challenges you are facing. Once your unique situation is understood, then you can determine what kinds of changes are needed.

Generally, this is done at the first meeting with the therapist. You will be asked a number of questions that, at first, may not seem too important. For example, the therapist is likely to ask, *"Why are you here?"* Or in the case of trying CBT through the pages of this book, ask yourself, *"Why are you reading this book?"* This will prompt you to do an internal examination of your motivation for wanting to try CBT.

You might also spend some time determining what your strengths are. While you are looking at CBT to solve many of your problems, you will use your strengths as a tool to combat your struggles. There are several ways you can uncover your strengths. These are usually the things that people tend to recognize and admire about you, those qualities that others appreciate about you. Maybe, at this point, you don't see these qualities in yourself, but others do, so consider talking to someone close to you to find out just what they see in you that can be useful.

Next, you will need to take a step back and examine how your life is going at the moment. But don't just do a surface look at the conditions. Take extra notice of how the anxiety/depression is affecting you. There are several different aspects that you can examine closely.

- **Relationships:** Relationships often affect our overall health probably more than anything else. When your marriage is on the skids, it usually means that you're not satisfied with your life in general and that attitude can lead to some very negative thoughts. However, if you have a life full of positive relationships and full of supportive people, your outlook on life will have a more positive spin.

  As you examine the relationships, look at how your anxiety/depression is affecting them. For example, you may have a supportive relationship, but is your depression causing you to pull away and not spend as much time with them. Your anxiety may be causing you to live your life on a short fuse, constantly snapping at them or keeping you angry and on edge all the time.

  Don't just look at a relationship with your spouse or significant other but consider how it is playing out with your parents, siblings, friends, children, and even coworkers. Determine what is good in your relationships and what is not. How do you feel about the people who have moved out of your life (either by moving away, a death, or an unresolved disagreement)?

  Finally, think about your relationships that are affecting your anxiety/depression. Are they making you more anxious or more depressed? Take note of the answer to these questions because you will have to face them later.

- **Physical Health:** Next, take some time to analyze your overall health. Here, you want to consider your eating habits, the amount of physical activity you're involved in, and what substances you regularly use (alcohol, drugs, etc.) The goal here is to draw a line between your regular habits and how they are affecting you physically. These can easily affect your moods and cause anxiety or depression.

As you consider health, think about any chronic health issues you're dealing with. Conditions like high blood pressure, diabetes, asthma, or other ongoing physical challenges can create huge inroads on your mood. If you're getting more physical exercise, how are you feeling about it? Do you enjoy your regular routine or do you find it a chore; something that you just have to get done? Is there a kind of activity that you enjoy more than others or do you just not like moving at all?

Look at how much alcohol or drugs you use each day. These include prescription drugs as well as less favorable ones. If you've had a problem with substance abuse in the past, this is something that you need to give some serious thought to.

The same weight should be given to your diet. If you are a stress eater, you are likely eating foods that are hampering your ability to function. You may not even realize that you're eating these foods. Another concern should be if you're eating enough or overeating. These habits will affect your weight, which could have a direct impact on your own self-image, self-esteem, and self-respect; all of which will affect your moods.

Sleep also can affect your physical health. If you're not getting enough or you're getting too much, it can have an impact on your daily routine. It can keep you from getting the kind of movement you need and even the kind of foods you eat. Look at any external factors that could be affecting your normal sleep routine: pets, partners, work, kids, etc.

All of us need to have some downtime. If we allow our lives to encroach on that time, our activity level will suffer. There are probably many things you'd like to be doing and many things you'd rather not be doing. If your activity level is too high, chances are that you haven't had much time to relax and destress. You may also not have had any time to do the kind of things you enjoy doing like sports, hobbies, travels, etc. You can be highly active and still not have time to do the things you enjoy.

You will take this week to examine your entire life to see how these factors and others are affecting your mood. Afterward, go back over everything you've noted and see how it affects you. First, look at how it has affected your life and your mood in the past, but then take some time to meditate on them. Note what negative emotions come out as you're doing this review. Common feelings that emerge just talking about these things include anxiety, joy, sorry, overwhelm, sad, melancholy, etc.

Setting Goals

With a better understanding of the problems you're coping with, it'll be much easier to set specific goals for you to start working towards. In CBT, goals need to be very specific, something that is measurable and within reach. You need to concentrate on the type of changes that will actually be meaningful to your life and that you feel you can reasonably achieve within a short amount of time.

It is important to not be vague at this point. Remember that CBT has a time limit. Whether the program you are on is six weeks or ten, your goals should reflect where you reasonably expect to be at that point. So, goals like "I want to be happier" or "I want to stop worrying so much," are not specific enough to maintain your motivation for the duration of the program.

Instead, your goals should have very defined parameters. "I want to be able to get up on time every day," or "I want to find time to do something I enjoy." Your goals need to relate directly to the specific problems you are facing. "I want to voice my opinion more in employee meetings."

You want to avoid making grand goals that will require a major commitment; instead, focus on something that is well within your ability to achieve in a one, two, or three-week period. When you make large goals that are far out of your scope of ability, try to set a series of smaller goals that will help you to reach the larger ones at a later date. You can have these larger expectations set for years later, but it's best to break them up into smaller steps with each one taking you closer and closer to what you ultimately want to achieve. As you progress through the program, you will develop a more balanced view of yourself, which will help you to improve in your ability to accomplish more.

Building Self-Esteem

When you are suffering from low self-esteem, CBT can be very practical in helping you to identify the source of your negative thoughts, and how it influences your behavior. By incorporating these strategies, those dealing with self-esteem issues can work their way towards a healthier lifestyle.

Because CBT works on your personal perception of yourself, the techniques learned will help you understand how your mind works to create its own meanings in your experiences, and then teach you how to reframe your negative views and alter them by focusing on building a more positive structure of thoughts to rely on.

Throughout your sessions, you may learn techniques like:

- **Cognitive Restructuring:** where you focus on thought patterns and their sources. By regular reflection on these patterns, you will learn how to analyze your method of judgment and start reshaping your perception into more realistic possibilities.

- **Behavioral Activation:** where you identify those situations that cause you discomfort or make you afraid. By engaging in this technique, you are encouraged to step out of your comfort zone and gradually learn how to insert yourself into new situations.

- **Assertiveness Training:** through assertiveness training, you learn to reclaim your self-confidence. Through this, you are motivated to step out of your area of comfort and assert yourself in various areas where you can build up your self-confidence.

- **Social Skills Training:** through this form of therapy, you learn to work on improving social skills. It may include learning how you interpret and analyze many of the social situations you may have to interact with. Since low self-esteem comes from a negative perception of interactions with others, learning how to interact in a variety of social environments will make you aware of how your mind processes these situations and redirects them into a more positive direction.

Anyone suffering from a low self-esteem can learn how their thoughts relate to their actions and how to reflect on their impact and work to redirect them in a healthier and more positive lifestyle.

Verbal Self-Talk

We talk to ourselves all the time, but when you have negative self-talk, it can be very damaging. We often say things to ourselves that we would never dare say to anyone else. Our stress does not just come from external input, but our own emotional makeup can significantly add to it. In fact, studies have shown that our emotional makeup can actually cause so much stress in our bodies that it changes our physical make-up. Negative self-talk can cause changes in a number of health issues including:

- Diarrhea/constipation
- Muscle tension and pain
- Ulcers
- Headaches
- Insomnia
- Teeth grinding
- High blood pressure
- Cold hands/feet

All of these, in addition to our anxiety and depression, we may be suffering from. Chronic stress depletes the body of the essential chemicals that it needs to function properly. When we lack these essentials, we leave ourselves open for a number of illnesses. However, it is possible for us to change the way we respond to external and internal elements and develop a more healing environment that will give us better health.

It starts with changing how we talk to ourselves. CBT can teach you how to control your negative reactions to different things by teaching you different ways to interpret your personal experiences. So, rather than berating yourself for a simple mistake, you could remind yourself of all the times you did things well.

This helps to reduce feelings of guilt, shame, and anxiety that are eroding our mental and physical health. By changing these negative thought patterns into positive affirmations, you will find your mental state will gradually begin to turn into another direction.

Counter Negative and Angry Feelings

Anger is a unique negative feeling. Unlike other negative emotions like sadness, guilt, or disgust, anger can also have a positive side to it, so all anger is not bad. Sometimes referred to as the moral emotion, it often appears in cases where morals are brought into question. Values like justice, fairness, and respect are at its core.

There may be times, however, when you may not be able to make the connection between the root of your anger and its actual cause. You may, for example, feel you are angry at one person or another, but the cause may be from an entirely different source. This makes anger a sort of an enigma. We know that it usually precedes aggression, so it pays to address this issue as soon as possible. Negative anger can be treated with several different approaches to CBT. In fact, studies show that in as little as 8-12 weeks, there have been some very promising results. Techniques such as problem-solving, relaxation strategies, and enhanced communication skills have all been very effective in helping people to handle their anger better.

Dealing With Feelings of Guilt

Everyone has to deal with guilt at some point. No matter who we are, holding onto the wrongs we've done in the past is probably the most common reason why people don't move forward. Most of it comes from having to deal with the consequences of the poor decisions we've made, but the feeling that one act can stop us from moving on with our lives can be crippling.

No matter what has been done in the past, since it is not possible to do those things over in a different way, when negative results occur, the guilt that results can become like a life sentence that you impose upon yourself. Getting rid of that guilt on your own can sometimes feel impossible.

Through CBT, you can be guided through looking at that past event and learn how to see it through fresh eyes; eyes that can see the situation from different angles. One particular technique applied is a technique called The Blame Pie. This tool helps you to see just how much control you had over the negative situation and that, in most cases, you were not totally responsible. It looks at each individual involved in the incident and divides the blame according to their contribution to the event. As each person is assigned a percentage of the blame, it literally lifts much of the weight off your shoulders.

This type of treatment, over time, can help someone to get past the weight of the responsibility they had and finally find themselves worthy of moving on to a better life.

Counteract Hopelessness

Sometimes, depression can become so deep that a person feels completely hopeless. Because depression is the result of negative thinking, recovery from something as severe as hopelessness can be painfully slow. Even if you have positive thoughts on occasion, when you reach the point of hopelessness, you may not allow them to surface long enough to reap the effects.

Normally, in a depressed state of mind, positive emotions are often squelched with more powerful, negative thoughts like "I don't deserve to be happy," or "I know this won't last." In their minds, even when they feel good, they are unable to enjoy it because they are waiting for the ax to fall.

Through CBT, identifying the pattern of thoughts that lead to negative behavior can be changed. Once you're better able to identify these patterns, you can recognize them when they arise, freeing your mind for more positive thoughts. This can be done in several phases:

- Identifying the problem and mapping out solutions.
- Write down more positive statements that can counteract the negative thoughts.
- Actively search for new opportunities to apply positive thoughts.
- Learn to accept disappointment as a normal part of life.

Chapter 6: Steps to Dealing with Mood Disorders and Depression

Preventing mood disorders and depression is at the heart of Cognitive Behavioral Therapy. It has a multilevel approach that starts small and builds, helping patients to change their thought processes in everything they do. With each step, they celebrate small advances that will help them to gradually get closer and closer to their goals.

The first phase of the therapy involves identifying the problem they are facing, which is generally the result of automatic and intrusive thoughts. This is a crucial phase of the therapy as it defines a starting point for the treatment needed. Without a solid knowledge of the problem, it would be difficult to target the right strategies and techniques to deal with it directly.

The second phase is a period of goal setting where they can work on where they want to be within a set timeframe. After identifying the biggest issues you may be facing, it is much easier to map out a series of steps that will help you to focus on the changes you want to make.

In phase three, you will need to identify the challenges and obstacles you will be facing that will likely get in the way of your goals. No path will be easy as you will have to deal with a variety of setbacks along the way. You can decide to use them as a roadblock preventing your progress, as an obstacle that will require you to make a detour on your path to success, or as a stepping stone used to help you to get to where you really want to be.

Phase four deals with learning how to challenge your automatic and intrusive thoughts. In this phase, patients learn how to separate reality from the exaggerated thoughts they normally have. Once these negative thoughts have been identified, they can be challenged by a series of questions that forces them to use logic to come to a more reasonable conclusion. At this point, you will need to look for factual evidence that will contradict your embedded beliefs. Once those beliefs have been identified and successfully refuted, then you can learn how to use the evidence to refute those beliefs. Over time, those beliefs will diminish and be replaced by more realistic ones.

Phase five helps with identifying even more automatic assumptions and beliefs. Now that the automatic thoughts have been identified, this phase takes it another step forward and isolates the deeper core beliefs that all people have. These are the ones that are more absolute and less flexible. They most likely have been formed in childhood, and unless changed, will stay with you throughout your life, getting reinforced over the years with each experience you have.

This phase is the best stage to address these issues because many of us are reluctant to accept that these thoughts are wrong until they have addressed their own automatic thoughts first. Challenging these beliefs is often like challenging who you are as a person because they have been deeply embedded in your mind for years to come.

Phase Six focuses on changing the behavior. Up until this point, all of the exercises are dealing with the cognitive activity in the mind. These changes can now begin to extend outward involving participation in different activities and events giving special attention to those that will deliver a more positive mood.

For those dealing with depression, participating in these activities is crucial to lifting the mood. In this phase, the focus should rely heavily on avoidance issues, depression, anxiety, and phobias. Its goal is to boost self-confidence so you are more comfortable engaging in more meaningful activities.

Phase Seven deals with the problem-solving strategies you will need. It brings home the main point of Cognitive Behavioral Therapy; convincing your mind that everything is all right and that any problems that come up, you are capable of handling. While challenging your negative thoughts and beliefs will produce good results, the ability to master the skills taught in the problem-solving phase will be the most effective in helping to ease behavioral issues.

It is important to note that each of these seven steps can help you to move closer to your goal, it will not work well for everyone. Those who are suffering from severe depression, emotional trauma, and those mental illnesses that are considered to be extreme won't likely be enough. Most of the exercises and strategies you learn in CBT can be done and practiced on your own, but if you're dealing with extreme emotional instability, then you may need more guided therapy to help you get back on the right path.

The problem-solving phase involves several steps:

1. Identify the problem and the specific elements you need to address.
2. Brainstorm possible solutions.
3. Evaluate each solution to determine the pros and cons of each.
4. Choose an optimal solution and then choose a backup.
5. Create a plan of action.
6. Execute the plan.
7. Review results and make needed adjustments.
8. If the problem is not resolved, start again at step 1.

At this phase, you will also need to review your lifestyle habits. Modifications will likely be necessary as an aid to improve how your brain processes thoughts. You will be coached in matters of sleep, eating, physical activity, and meditation.

Most people will see impressive results after applying these methods over a period of several weeks. The most common approach is to take one or two weeks to address each step. After you have successfully met the challenges of one phase, then do not hesitate to move on to the next one. Hesitation could interrupt the momentum you've developed and could cause you to lose your steam.

Chapter 7: Multimodal Model

As you can see, there are multiple ways that CBT can help a person to counteract their negative tendencies. With their Multimodal strategy, the technique gets a little more in-depth with a closer look at the seven different aspects of the human personality.

With this model, therapy consists of using a variety of models at one time, all of which are able to be adapted to many situations because they are completely interactive. They also share the same core beliefs that an individual will use to build his thought processes on. They consist of a combination of several elements including:

- Their Biological and genetic makeup
- The Effects of their experiences
- The Sensations that exist between thoughts, feelings, and behavior
- The Imagery that occurs in their own minds, mental images both negative or positive
- Their Cognition, or the way they think whether positive or negative
- Their Interpersonal relationships with others
- Their Drugs/biology, or their physical experiences, or the use of substances

These are considered the core of this type of therapy. They can be easily identified with the acronym BASIC ID. Each of these modalities is used to help narrow down the areas in which the coaching sessions should focus on.

The beauty of the Multimodal Model is that it recognizes that different people will respond to different modalities. You may be capable of handling your problems on your own while others will rely heavily on the support of others, and others may prefer to deal with their problems through certain activities. All of these can be incorporated into the seven areas of the BASIC ID, so it is possible to focus on those strategies that will allow them to overcome the problems they face in a manner that they can feel more comfortable with.

The goal of MMD is to help the individual make the necessary changes so they can make the transition from their current state of mind to a more progressive and adaptable mental state. MMD is often used in highly complex cases of depression and performance anxiety. Those who benefit the most are experiencing negative behavior so extreme that their lives are paralyzed to the point that they are unable to move forward. Their careers and their families are already at risk or on the verge of falling apart. Some have a level of fear that has reached a climax that it has had a heavy impact on nearly all seven of the modalities, and an intervention is likely the only possible solution.

Its success can be attributed to the principle that by approaching several issues at the same time, an individual may find themselves dependent on substances or other crutches to deal with them. It could be a combination of health problems, emotional issues, and financial distress all at the same time. Each case severe enough to be addressed on their own but through MMD, it is possible to address all of these issues at the same time to facilitate a speedier recovery.

The Seven Modalities You Should Know About

Because most psychological problems tend to be multifaceted, it is necessary to start by understanding each of the seven modalities that are actually affecting you. When you consider that many of the intervention techniques that people naturally turn to are substances, it is helpful to give even more consideration to the last modality, drugs or substances, as they will hold many techniques that can reveal your inner self. Now, let's take a closer look at each one of them to see how they are used in CBT.

Behavior: This aspect of MMD takes a close look at everything a patient does. This includes his habits, gestures, actions, etc. Some of his behaviors will be healthy while others will not be. Unhealthy behaviors that require particular attention could be those that are destructive, immoral, childish, illegal, impulsive, controlling, or otherwise, inappropriate.

Most patients will seek therapy because their unwanted behaviors are causing problems in their lives. Practices such as overeating, excessive drinking, hoarding, rebellion, self-mutilation, etc. are the most common. The goal is to change the behavior itself through techniques like modeling, desensitization, and aversive conditioning. The trick is that nearly all unwanted behaviors are connected to the other modalities as well, so by including this in the MMD therapy sessions, there is a much higher chance of success and the prevention of a relapse.

Affect: This modality refers to the inner feelings and emotions you are experiencing. Throughout the process, you may feel a wide range of emotions, but the focus of the therapy is to address the feelings you don't like. So, while you may feel happy, sad, afraid, frustrated, and bored, the sessions will likely involve the negative emotions first. Many who are seeking therapy for other reasons will often find that these emotions are at the root of their problems, even if they don't realize it in the beginning. The negative emotions are usually the underlying trigger for a wide range of other feelings that are often buried deep inside.

Sensation: We have five senses – sight, hearing, touch, taste, and smell, which contribute to all of our physiological experiences. Negative sensations may be butterflies in the stomach, tense muscles, physical pain, rapid heartbeat, headaches, cold hands or feet, sweating, nausea, skin crawling, and shortness of breath. Some more extreme sensations could also be hallucinations and/or illusions.

Imagery: This modality consists of the mental images that are built up in a

190

person's mind. It includes things they may fantasize about, their daydreams, and their own personal self-image. Common in those who suffer from anxiety disorders, their fears are part of their imagery. They also have an excessive worry about the future. Those who struggle with depression may have images that are extremely negative and distorted, far from the reality of things. Addressing one's imagery will help them to learn how to adjust the view of the world and give them a more realistic and accurate view.

Cognition: Focuses on a person's beliefs, attitudes, and judgments. When thoughts are negative like limiting or distorted beliefs about something, they can contribute significantly to depression, anxiety, or any number of other disorders. When a person believes they are not worthy of something, it can have an impact on their relationships, employment, and other areas of their life, which can be very damaging.

Interpersonal Relationships: This takes a closer look at how they interact with others, their social skills, how they relate to people, and what kind of support system they have or is missing in their lives. A close look at their relationships will reveal if they know how to develop and maintain a lasting relationship, feel connected to others, and if they have a good balance in mental health. Those getting over a breakup, needing to resolve conflict, or are antisocial will usually find that they are also lacking in the areas of effect and cognition as well.

Drugs, Health, Biology: This is a combination of several things. First, it includes a person's physical health. Whether he has been fighting off any serious illnesses, his overall physical condition, any physical limitations, his age, or chronic pain are just some of the health concerns they may have. It will also include biological factors like his genetics and brain chemistry and his need for medical treatment or medications. Finally, this modality looks at his lifestyle habits including diet and nutrition, activity level, sleep and eating habits, smoking, and drug and alcohol use. Close attention needs to be considered when dealing with substances. Few people realize just how much of an impact these habits can have on your mood or mental state. By evaluating this factor carefully, you may be surprised at what it can reveal.

There are two ways these seven modalities can be assessed. It is either with a one-on-one interview with a therapist or by filling out a Multimodal Life History Inventory questionnaire. Once an assessment is determined based on the BASIC ID, then a program of therapeutic techniques and strategies can be implemented starting with the modality that represents the biggest problem.

Chapter 8: Rational Emotive Behavioral Therapy

Rational Emotive Behavioral Therapy (REBT) places most of its importance on the thought processes of an individual. Like all other forms of CBT, it is based on the same premise that what we think triggers our feelings, which in turn, will trigger our behavior. The main idea behind REBT is to help those people who view their personal experiences in a negative way. However, they do not address the experience directly. Instead, the behavior is adjusted based on how they "perceived" the experience.

Through REBT, patients are taught how to challenge their own beliefs and replace them with a more accurate line of reasoning. It targets the inner beliefs, so they can deal with their experiences in a more realistic way. When successful, it can be very powerful, changing not just the way one thinks but also their perception of life in general.

REBT works because it recognizes that logic is not always an effective part of the human psyche. Even with logic, it is not always the best way to solve problems. Computers operate entirely on logic to perform their functions; they absorb data, analyze it, and using logic determine an acceptable output. The human brain, however, processes information differently, often without the use of logic. Therefore, some of their conclusions can be far removed from reality.

The focus of Rational Emotive Therapy is to teach people to think in a more logical manner. It works to break down the instinctual thinking process by using logical reasoning to interfere with the irrational assumptions they are making. Once these irrational thoughts have been replaced with more positive ones, it will start to filter down and change the inappropriate behavior to actions that are more positive.

No matter what negative thought a person may have, its roots are often deep within an unrealistic world. To combat this type of reasoning, REBT applies something called the ABCDE model of thinking.

A: Activating Event

An inciting event is identified which triggers the irrational belief. This could be any number of negative experiences including an argument with someone, a car accident, or the loss of a job. It is the trauma of this event that compels the mind to create a new irrational thought or belief.

B: The Belief

Once the belief has been created, the mind will automatically revisit it every time a similar negative event occurs. Each time the mind goes back to the belief, it is reinforced causing the person to get stuck in a spiral of negative behavior without ever really understanding why it happened in the first place.

C: Consequences

The belief will trigger the consequences of their irrational thoughts. Some consequences could be emotional as in the case of guilt or shame, while others could be behavioral as in overeating or some form of substance abuse. The underlying emotions for these behaviors could be depression, lack of self-confidence, or hostility.

D: Dispute

The dispute phase of the program is when you learn to challenge that belief system and see it as irrational. You begin to recognize it as the root of your problems. At this stage, you learn to argue with your subconscious mind and dispute your negative beliefs. You will be asked to come up with convincing proof that will successfully contradict your imprinted way of thinking.

E: Effect

You could also call this phase reinforcement. Once you have had your internal debate and successfully convinced yourself that your irrational belief is wrong, more positive behaviors will be much easier to come by. You'll feel a stronger self-esteem, you'll be bolder, or you'll just feel a lot better overall.

In most cases, REBT can be done without the aid of a therapist. This model can help anyone get to the root of their negative behavior and arm them with the tools they need to change. It motivates people to look deeply at how their thoughts are developed and how to apply rationale to their beliefs and replace negative thoughts with a more realistic view that will build them up rather than tearing them down.

Chapter 9: Dialectical Behavior Therapy

Dialectical Behavior Therapy is more like a positive form of psychotherapy that can be tailored to treat those with some form of borderline personality disorder.

More like a form of "talk therapy," DBT focuses on the psychosocial elements of treatment. Its theory is based on the premise that some people's behavior is so extreme that their reaction to romantic, familial, or social relationships is a manner that is far removed from the norm.

Those who fall into this category experience emotional extremes where their arousal levels can happen very quickly and their emotions are at such a peak that the reactions are at a very high level, taking them much longer to return to normal after an episode. They generally see things only in black or white with extreme emotional outbursts that can leave quite a bit of damage in their wake.

Because of this, they find themselves falling into one problem after another with no internal ability to manage their emotions. Therefore, they get no relief when their emotions spiral out of control. DBT is made up of three different elements:

Support-Oriented: Identifying their strengths and learning how to use them to help them feel better about themselves.

Cognitive-Based: Identifying the negative thought patterns and finding new ways to cope with triggering events so that their lives are more stable.

Collaborative: Rooting out underlying problems by working through assignments, active role-play, and learning self-soothing practices, so they can manage their own outbursts.

Through each of these sessions, the focus will be on two primary components:

1. **Structured Individual Psychotherapy Sessions**

Working with a therapist in a one-on-one session, patients will learn problem-solving behavior and openly discuss very specific issues that may have occurred in the past. These challenges could be anything from suicidal tendencies to self-mutilation. The more serious the issue, the more priority it should be given when working with the therapist. Minor issues may be assigned for the patient to deal with as homework.

During these sessions, you may also learn certain behaviors that can be applied to interrupt the negative habits. This adaptive behavior will have an emphasis on helping you to manage your emotions in the face of trauma much better. The objective here is to work towards a more socially acceptable behavior, so you can have better relationships with others.

2. Group Therapy Sessions

In group therapy, patients work their way through four different modules where they are taught practical skills they can rely on to help them cope with their negative patterns. Each skill has its own unique quality that can be used to minimize the negativity in their heads.

Mindfulness: A form of meditation where patients are helped to be more aware of their circumstances and the triggers that are causing their behaviors. Through mindfulness, they are taught how to observe, describe, and participate in their own thought processes as a neutral party. Then, with the use of special exercises, they learn how to recognize the triggers in their own mind, so they are better able to manage those reactions.

Interpersonal Effectiveness: Through practice sessions, they learn how to interact with others in a variety of scenarios. The process they go through is very similar to what is taught in many assertiveness training programs. Each session focuses on specific strategies to employ when getting to where they can ask for what they need, refuse things they don't, and specific coping mechanisms for when they are dealing with conflict.

Distress Tolerance: With distress tolerance, patients are given better ways to cope with disappointing and distressing circumstances. They learn how to accept things in a nonjudgmental manner. Rather than focusing on the negative, they will be better able to deal with real life situations that happen without their approval. Through this module, they are prepared with self-soothing techniques and other coping mechanisms that will reduce negative emotions and behavior.

Emotional Regulation: Learning how to regulate emotions is the key to managing negative behavior. Through the emotion regulation module, patients learn how to recognize the signs of oncoming intense emotions and use their coping strategies to manage them better. In this phase, they will be expected to address different emotional aspects including:

- Properly identifying and labeling their emotions when they arise.
- Recognizing the common obstacles that have been getting in the way of changing negative emotions.
- Lowering their susceptibility to negative emotions.
- Developing strategies to create more positive emotional experiences.
- Techniques that allow them to use their mindfulness to enhance positive emotions.
- They will also learn how to suppress their natural tendency long enough to choose another behavioral option opposite of what their instincts will do.
- They are given strategies they can utilize in distressful situations that will boost their tolerance levels.

With DBT, there are two main components, but because those that need CBT are most likely dealing with behavioral issues, they will focus most of their lessons in a group therapy environment, so they are able to practice their new skills and strategies they will need when interacting with others. DBT is still a relatively new program, but even so, it has already received recognition as a gold standard method of psychological treatment.

PART V

Chapter 1: Energy Healing- The Key to Holistic Health

Understanding the impacts of energy imbalances and corresponding physical, mental, spiritual health

How many times have you, or another adult in your life, said the words "I just don't have the energy I used to have."? Most adults know the feeling of looking at the energy children have as they run about, enjoying life, exploring their surroundings, and never seeming to grow tired. Many of us are left reflecting back on the distance past when we, too, had such energy, and wondering where it went.

From the time children enter school, they begin to be presented with expectations. Stand in a straight line, raise your hand, don't talk while the teacher is talking. Each year, the level of responsibility and expectation seems to increase. While rules, regulations, and individual responsibility are important for a functioning society, there are numerous expectations and social pressures put on people as they grow which can be incredibly harmful.

It is generally around middle school when children become more acutely aware of their bodies and societal beauty standards which tell them what they "should" look like. Children are likely to become aware of the trends, such as which clothes the "cool kids" are wearing. The endless battle to feel like enough begins, and can lead to a plethora of issues with self-esteem, eating disorders, and mental illness. In addition to the basic societal pressures to be accepted and considered attractive, many children are also faced with difficult situations at home where their own needs are not being met, they are having to provide for and protect themselves in the only ways they know how, avoid abusive parents, care for younger siblings, or worry about if they'll have anything to eat that day. Even if children have a relatively healthy home life, this is the age when they will begin to become aware of the issues that plague their family (every family has issues) whether this is divorce, an alcoholic parent, the death of a pet or loved one, etc.

We live in a society which thrives off of consumerism. We are flooded with images of how the next vacation, new pair of shoes, nicer car, nicer house, or perfect partner will make us happy, and all of the things we need to change about ourselves in order to fulfill those things. Eventually, all the energy we had as a child starts going towards maintaining our image in society, trying to have all the "best" life has to offer (which always happens to be everything we do not have), and attempting to be as "successful" as possible in the eyes of society and other people. With no time to rest in the present moment, recharge, and appreciate what we already have, it is no wonder so many of us are completely drained of energy. In such a fast-paced society that discourages breaks, our energy will become depleted and we will find ourselves thrown out of balance and unable to obtain true happiness and well-being. Overtime, this depletion and imbalance can lead to a sense of spiritual disconnection, extreme mental health issues, and an increased risk of physical pain, illness, and even earlier death.

Chapter 2: Energy Healing and Overcoming Suffering

Energy and Grief/Trauma

Every human being knows that loss is a natural part of life. The one certain thing in life is that we, and everyone we know, is going to die. However, in such a fast-paced society, we are often given a very short grace period before being expected to swallow our grief and "move on" when we lose those closest to us. It is not abnormal for people to receive a bereavement period of only a few days before being expected to be back in the classroom or office and be fully functional. There is very little space for the grief journey, and most people are expected to harbor their feelings and keep their grief to themselves.

The grief process is expansive and incredibly energy draining. When we don't receive the adequate support from those around us, or adequate space to heal, our body begins to break down piece by piece. The empty spaces within us will swallow us up into states of depression, numbness, isolation, and pure exhaustion. Just like a wound being denied the correct treatment and care, the wounds of unresolved grief will fester and leave us feeling completely drained of energy and vitality for life.

Unresolved trauma also has an incredibly destructive impact on the body. Trauma can occur as a result of grief itself, as well as emotional or domestic abuse, accident or illness, war, sexual assault, childhood maltreatment, etc. The body holds trauma in various places, and the brain switches over from the logical ability to discern safety and danger into an easily triggered emotional state. An overactive emotional brain loses the ability to think clearly, make decisions, and recognize threats. People who have unresolved trauma are likely to be easily triggered and deal with unexplained outbursts of anger, fear, relationship issues, reckless behavior, and health problems. When trauma sits in the body unresolved, the brain is unable to understand that the traumatic event has ended. Therefore, it will stay in a consistent fight-or-flight state, which is incredibly draining and will leave the body with no energy. Not only will trauma victims experience low energy levels, they will also experience severe issues maintaining positive relationships and overall well-being.

Energy and Mental Health

There are numerous factors which can contribute to mental health issues.

As previously discussed, societal issues and unresolved grief and trauma can yield higher levels of anxiety, depression, and PTSD. It is also very common for people to suffer from mood disorders, personality disorders, disordered eating, substance abuse, etc. The list is long for psychological ailments and how they happen, and it has been proven that 1 in 3 people will be diagnosed with a mental illness in their lifetime. Even without a specific disorder, most people will have periods of life where their mental health suffers greatly.

No matter what a person's struggle with mental health looks like, or what they are doing (or not doing) in terms of treatment, the body expends a lot of energy when a part of it is unwell.

Daily Energy Regulation

No matter what it is in your life that is causing you to feel depleted, it is vital to pay attention to the energy fields within the body and identify the areas of greatest pain and imbalance. In the spectrum of health, people often take measures such as going to see the doctor, therapist, or grief counselor, taking medication, and making lifestyle changes such as finding a hobby or increasing exercise. However, a piece that is commonly overlooked in the healing journey is healing energetically. No matter how much you invest in your mental, physical, emotional, and spiritual health, if your energies remain imbalanced, it is impossible to reach a state of full wellness. That being said, energy healing is the missing piece in most people's quests for holistic health.

In many cases, it can be beneficial to seek the help of energy healers, massage therapists, and reiki, craniosacral therapy, or bodywork practitioners. These practitioners are trained in getting in touch with your energy centers and helping bring them back into balance through healing touch, body movements, and visualization techniques. If you are dealing with energy imbalance, seeing a practitioner can be an excellent investment in unlocking your highest levels of health and joy in life.

It is also possible to use a variation of the body scan mediation from chapter 3 to check in with your energy levels on your own. By taking notice of the sensations in each area of your body, you can come closer in touch with any area of your body where you experience regular pain, tension, or other unpleasant feelings. This is often a sign of imbalance or trapped energy. Additionally, the tense and release technique in each area of the body can yield healing and balance by releasing negative energy and tension. It is important to check in with yourself daily, asking your body where energy may be trapped or depleted and what you can do to replenish yourself.

Chapter 3: The Daily Energy Healing Journey

Understanding Your Energy Field: Daily Energy Healing

Meditation with Journaling (Week 5)

There is great variety when it comes to human energy fields. People experience varying levels of sensitivity to the energy of other people and the environment. Some people are incredibly in tune with "vibes", others are empaths who feel the emotional experiences of others on a deep level, while still others experience very little of either. There is also a lot of variation in the way people recharge energetically, as well as what depletes them. In the common case of introverts and extroverts, for example, introverts need time alone to replenish their energy and feel balanced, while extroverts recharge in stimulating environments with other people around. One of the first steps to protecting your personal energetic field is to understand how it works.

Understanding Your Energy Field Journal Prompt (Week 5):

When you feel exhausted and not like yourself, which activities are most likely to replenish your energy? Do you enjoy a night out with friends? Yoga? A walk in the park? Leisure reading? Finding a new adventure? Taking a bubble bath? Listening to your favorite music on blast? List 5-10 activities which help you gain balance and feel energized.

Now, make a list of the things that make you feel most drained. These can be large things, like a specific task at your job, or small things like doing the dishes. You may find that you feel drained if you spend too much time alone or, consequently, when you spend too much time around other people.

When it comes to activities that make you feel drained, ask yourself to what extent that specific thing is necessary in your life. If you find yourself feeling drained from spending too much time around other people, for example, you can easily make a change by scheduling more "nothing time" or "alone time" into your days and taking the time you need to replenish. Household tasks and daily responsibilities are necessary, but by being aware of the ones that drain you the most, you can bring more attention into the process and doing what you need to replenish energy before or after.

Protecting Your Energy Field: Daily Energy Healing Meditation with Journaling (Week 6)

Close your eyes and ask yourself "what does my energy field look like?" Write down any specific colors, textures, shapes, or patterns of movement.

Once you have an image in your mind of your energy field, ask yourself "What does it look like for outside energies to enter my field?" Write down what healthy and unhealthy outside energies look like.

Then ask yourself "How can I regulate the energies entering my field? What does it look like when I decide what I will let in?" Describe this process.

Finally, ask yourself "How does my body feel when I regulate what I allow to enter my energy field?" Write down everything that comes to mind.

Healing Through Trapped Emotion Release: Daily Energy Healing Meditation with Journaling (Week 7)

In our society, we are often faced with life circumstances that force us to repress our basic human emotions. It is very possible for anger, rage, or grief to become stuck in the body because it is considered "impractical" to have those reactions in public. Similarly, we often hear about people being described as "annoyingly happy" or "overly emotional." Most of us are taught not only to manage our emotions, but to distance ourselves from them and react emotionally only in certain contexts. Additionally, we tend to suppress negative emotions such as fear, shame, inadequacy, and insecurity, for the purpose of appearing like we have everything together. Between life events and societal expectations, it is very easy for the emotions we suppress to become trapped in our bodies, which can create adverse health effects, negatively impact our relationships, and keep us from living our best lives.

Begin by making a list of as many emotions as you can think of

Run down the list of emotions one by one, asking yourself "Is there anywhere in my body I am holding *particular emotion*?"

Write down the emotions you feel are trapped. Take some time to journal about how certain emotions arose, or times when you felt you had to suppress your emotions.

With each emotion you have labeled as being trapped, write: "I give myself permission to release this *particular emotion*

Cultivating Self-Trust in your Healing Journey: Daily Energy Healing Meditation with Journaling (Week 8)

No matter what you do in your life, there will always be people who don't understand the choices you make, or who judge the path you are on. When it comes to renewing and protecting your energy, there is no room for anyone else's opinions or emotions in regards to your journey. It requires a great deal of self-trust to go your own way and let what other people think about it roll off your back. For this reason, it is vital to begin everyday establishing a sense of self-trust with your own journey and energy management skills. The following four journal questions will help you direct your energy before going about your day.

What are you most grateful for today?

What are your intentions for how you will direct your energy today?

What are your fears/things you perceive as a potential threat?

What are your commitments to yourself and the world?

Mini Meditation Toolbox: 25 Quick and Easy Energy Restoration and Protection Meditations

One-Minute Energy Cleanse

- This meditation is useful if you find yourself with a person or in a specific situation that feels negative or energetically draining. You do not need to be alone to complete this meditation

- Pause where you are and allow yourself to take a few deep, cleansing breaths

- Focus exclusively on your breathing; you may close your eyes or leave them open

- Feel the inner power within the core of your body, around your abdomen. Remind yourself that you are in control and have the power to maintain balance.

- As you inhale, pull love, light, and peace into your body

- As you exhale, breathe out pain, annoyance, and toxicity

- Begin by entering a space in nature. This can be on the beach, in the mountains, near a river, in a garden, by the lake, or in your own yard

- If possible, slip your shoes off so your bare feet are in contact with the earth

- Start with a few cleansing breaths, taking note of everything you see, hear, smell, and feel in your environment

- Placing the soles of your feet on the ground, begin to breathe, pulling the energy from the earth up through your body

- Remember that you are One with the nature that courses around you. Allow it to heal what is broken within you and leave you feeling rejuvenated

Re-Centering Head Hold (3-5 minute meditation)

- Close your eyes and place the palm of one hand horizontally across the crown of your head, and the other palm across your forehead (over the energetic points of the Crown and Third Eye chakras). This position can be done while standing, sitting, or lying down.

- While clutching your head in this position, bring attention to any sensations in your body. What needs your attention most right now?

- Allow yourself to come back to the present moment, feeling grounded in your body and in your experience

- Breathe in awareness, focus, and comfort, exhaling anxiety and distraction

- When you open your eyes, notice how you feel grounded in your space

- This meditation is useful for energy protection before going out in to the world, whether that is to work, the supermarket, an appointment, etc.

- Although you do not know what kinds of energies you may encounter, or which people may try to take your energy from you, remind yourself that you are in control of your own energy and that you have the capacity to protect yourself

- Close your eyes and imagine a dark-blue, almost black cloak made of soft, thick material like a velvet night sky. The cloak is full-length with a hood to protect all of your chakras.

- Imagine a ray of light outlining the cloak in whatever color(s) feel most magical, protective, and authentic to who you are

- Set off into the world knowing that you are safe within yourself and your energy cloak, and that you do not need to be afraid

- When energy is lacking or out of balance, the spaces we live in are likely to reflect that imbalance with clutter and messiness. The more we feel like we "don't have our lives together", the more likely we are to have a messy desk, dishes piling up in the sink, laundry that still needs to be folded, or a car that has not been cleared of trash

- Such spaces do not allow for peace and mental clarity, and can be even more draining to come back to after a long day

- Dedicate yourself to one area of your life to de-clutter. This can be your kitchen, your car, your bedroom, etc. Close your eyes before beginning and take a few deep, cleansing breaths to approach the task calmly

- Begin to address all of the clutter in the space, not only picking it up, but putting it into a designated area where it can be organized and easy to find

- You may find that you want to create a special shelf or move some furniture around to make the space less cluttered. As you go, notice the energy that continues to unfold in your body

- When you finish, place a "clutter basket" in your room, the car, the living room, etc. where you can compile all the clutter throughout the day and put it away before bed

De-Cluttering your Mind (5-minute meditation)

- Close your eyes and begin to breathe deeply

- Ask yourself "What is taking up the most space in my mind right now?"

- Bring your attention to whatever it is that is distracting you, and why it makes you feel out of control

- Breathe into that situation, saying "I have control over this situation, and I am not going to let it spill out into the rest of my day. I am clearing this space."

- This meditation is ideal to perform in the morning, or before going out to interact with the world or other people

- Sit in a place where you feel energized (on the porch, in your meditation corner, etc.)

- Close your eyes and begin to breathe, checking in with any unresolved emotions or senses within the body

- Now begin to picture your energy field. Say to yourself: "My energy field is my sacred space, and other energies will only permeate it when I allow them to."

- Breathe into this thought for several moments

- Now, bring this thought into your mental space: "I have the wisdom to discern what belongs to me and what belongs to other people. I can be empathetic and attentive to other people's emotions, struggles, and opinions, without assuming responsibility for them."

- Begin by selecting your favorite scented Epsom salts. You may also customize your bath with petals, oils, and candles as according to the healing plants, herbs, and oils listed in Chapter 4

- Run a hot bath, letting your Epsom salts and other elements saturate the water

- Customize your space with the light of candles, meditative music, and anything else that makes you feel at peace

- Find a comfortable position inside the tub. Close your eyes, and feel your entire body relax into the heat and gentle movement of the water.

- Begin to conduct a body scan, feeling entirely vulnerable to this moment at peace with only yourself

- Ask your body "What do I need right now?"

- The water should be hot enough that you begin to sweat (be sure to have a glass of water nearby). As you sweat, imagine your body purging itself of every blockage, every impurity, and every negativity

- Close your eyes and begin to breathe

- Bring the image of your energy field to your mind. You may picture a wall, a bubble, or a glowing ring of light (this image may also differ depending on the day)

- Picture what other energies look like, floating around your field like particles in an atom. Say to yourself "I am in control of what comes in."

- Imagine yourself recognizing people who are trying to take your energy or bear their burdens. Imagine any fear, anger, or resentment you may feel.

- Say to yourself "No, not today." Imagine your bubble becoming impermeable, your wall being sealed, your glowing ring of light rejecting anything that does not belong inside

- Allow yourself to feel empowered over your energy, without feeling any resentment or judgment towards those who once posed a threat

Building your Sanctuary

- Sit down and close your eyes, beginning to breathe into yourself

- With each breath, ask yourself "What makes me feel safe?" Repeat three times.

- Switch the phrase to "What makes me feel at peace?" Repeat three times.

- Switch the phrase to "What makes me feel loving?" Repeat three times

- Switch to "What makes me feel joy?"

- Lastly, ask yourself "What makes me feel renewed?"

- When you ask yourself these questions, you may see certain crystals, scenes in nature, types of music, plants, aromas, decorations, activities, or color schemes. Take note of whatever comes to mind.

- Use these things that come to you in meditation to mindfully cultivate a space for yourself to come into every day when you need time to recharge. This can be a meditation corner, a spot in the backyard, or any other space that is sacred to you and provides feelings of security and rest.

Cultivating Non-Reaction

- This meditation can be used when encountering a stressful situation, having a difficult conversation, or otherwise entering a state of nervous or angry energy

- Before responding to whatever the negative stimulant is, breathe into the moment. Close your eyes if needed.

- Tell yourself "I can choose not to expend energy on this interaction. I can choose to move peacefully into the next moment."

- Feel the tension within you melt away as you make the choice not to internalize the stress of the situation or the negative energy coming at you

Boundary Setting

- Find a quiet place to sit and self-reflect. Breathe into the moment

- After you have settled into your breath, ask yourself "What people, circumstances, or tasks drain my energy and leave me feeling agitated or exhausted?"

- Allow the answers to rise into your consciousness at will. Meditate on every name, every task, every circumstance which makes you feel tense and throws your energy out of balance.

- With each name, circumstance, and task, say to yourself "This *person, place, thing* has no power over me. I can maintain my energy in spite of it."

- Next, ask yourself "Where do I need to draw the line with this *person, place, thing*?"

- Listen to your intuition tell you what your boundaries should be. Perhaps, this looks like gently cutting off a toxic person, or limiting your interaction time with them. It could be quitting a job that is no longer good for you, or asking for accommodations to make your environment more positive. It could be telling someone who expects you to bear their burdens that their energies are no longer your responsibility. Or, perhaps it is to establish a self-care activity to do directly after a draining task.

- If your energy has ever been thrown out of balance by trauma, there are likely still factors of your environment which can strike at any time, causing your body to react in the same way it did at the time of the trauma.

- Breathe into the moment, asking yourself "what elements of my environment cause me to lose control of my logic and feel afraid, helpless, irrational, in pain, or otherwise unbalanced or unhealthy energetically"

- These elements are called "triggers." Bring your awareness to these triggers, simply allowing them to be there without judgment.

- Say to yourself "that moment in time is over. I can now release myself."

- Begin by determining 3-5 affirmations or manifestations for the day ahead ("I manifest peace," "I am content," "I am present," "I manifest energy," "I am growing," "I manifest healing," "I manifest loving-kindness", etc.)

- Breathe deeply, pondering the affirmations/manifestations

- Choose your first manifestation/affirmation. With your index and middle fingers on both hands, begin tapping lightly on the crown of your head, repeating the manifestation or affirmation three times

- Move to the temples, tapping and saying the manifestation/affirmation three times

- Repeat at the inner corners of the brow bone

- Repeat just above the brow line

- Repeat at the top of the cheek bones

- Repeat below the ear lobes at the crest of the jawbone

- Repeat at the top of the chest

- Repeat on the left wrist, then switch to right wrist

- Switch to the next affirmation/manifestation and go through the process again, staying in touch with your breath throughout

Listening to your Intuition

- Find a space where you feel completely comfortable and relaxed

- Begin to breathe deeply, coming into the present moment

- Ask yourself "What does my inner self need me to know right now?"

- Keep breathing, holding space for whatever answer arises

- If necessary, you can ask follow-up questions to yourself like "Is there any threat I need to be prepared to protect myself from?" or "How can I best love the world today?" Or "What do I need to do to take care of myself today?"

- Continue to breathe and hold space, trusting that your heart will guide you to make the correct decisions for yourself

Memory Reclamation (specifically for healing of trauma victims)

- Find a space where you feel totally safe and undisturbed. It is best to do this meditation on a day where you can invest in self-care and rest.

- Begin to breathe, telling yourself "I am safe. I am safe. I am safe."

- Allow the memory of a particularly traumatic event to come to your mind. Continue to breathe, telling yourself "I am safe."

- Pay attention to the details of that memory. What do you see? What do you hear? What do you feel?

- As the memory progresses, allow it to release its energetic hold on your body. Tell yourself "That was then. This is now. I am safe."

- Feel the trauma release its hold on you, restoring itself to a basic memory of the past

Defining your Needs

- Sit in a peaceful place, breathing into the moment

- Bring attention to any pain or unrest within your body. Without judgment, allow it to be there, asking if there is anything you should learn from it.

- Generally, where there is pain or unrest, there is a need being left unmet. Ask yourself "What is it that I need?"

- Allow your needs to arise into your consciousness ("I need a day off for my mental health," "I need a trip into nature," "I need a bath," "I need a warm, nourishing meal," "I need to go to sleep early," etc.)

- Breathe into each need, envisioning yourself meeting that particular need

- Ask yourself "Is there anyone else I need to make aware of these needs?"

- Envision yourself having a calm conversation about your needs with your boss, your partner, your family, or a friend. Envision them reacting gently and yourself feeling better understood and supported.

- Continue to breathe into your capacity to meet your energetic needs and make those needs known to others.

"Nothing Time"

- Set aside a minimum of one hour of time with absolutely nothing scheduled

- Sit down, breathing into the moment. Tell yourself "this is my time. I have nowhere to be, nothing to do, I do not need to feel rushed."

- Allow your deepest intuition to guide your next step. Do whatever comes to mind first

- While you proceed with your "nothing time", allow your breath to guide every move

Discovering your Support System

- Bring your attention to the present moment, focusing on your breath

- Ask yourself "Who of the people I know understands and embraces me for who I truly am?"

- Breathe with each name that comes up, allowing loving-kindness and appreciation for that person to flow through your body

- Ask yourself "Who in my life encourages me to reach my full potential?

- Repeat the action of breathing with each name that arises

- Ask yourself "Who in my life do I feel most at rest with?"

- Repeat the action of breathing with each name that arises

- Continue to breathe, saying to yourself "These are my people. This is my support system. I will allow myself to lean on them when I need to."

Glowing Love-Energy

- Find a restful position and begin to breathe

- Imagine the aura of your energy field. How big is it? What color is it?

- Say to yourself "I am pure love. I have room to love the entire universe and everything in it."

- Continue to repeat this phrase with every breath. Picture the aura expanding and glowing brighter

Jaguar Spirit Animal Protection

- Bring yourself into the present moment with deep breathing

- From the depth of your being, say "I call on the spirit of the jaguar to protect me."

- Feel the reverberations of the jaguar's protection through your body, aiding you in repelling negative energy and toxicity

- Imagine a fierce, beautiful guard of your energy field, encircling you with fierce love and security

Energetic Breathing (1-3-minute meditation)

- Take some space away from your everyday life (in the bathroom, in the car, etc.) to just breathe

- Implement the 5-5-7 breathing technique

- With every breath in, say to yourself, "I breathe in pure energy."

- With every breathe out, say to yourself, "I breathe out *exhaustion, *toxicity, *negativity, etc."

- Continue until you feel the tingle of pure energy coursing through your veins

Energetic Dancing/Movement

- Find a space where you can be alone and feel completely secure

- Play a song that stirs your soul and emotions, causing you to have a visceral reaction in the body each time you hear it

- As the song begins, close your eyes and deep breathe, maybe swaying back and forth slightly

- When you feel ready, release your body to move as it feels led. No choreography, no expectations, simply letting the movement of the moment lead your body into a state of pure surrender and release

- Surrender entirely to the moment, trusting your body to release any tension or trauma

- Give your body the space and freedom to heal, coming into energetic harmony

The Art of Saying "No"

- Close your eyes and begin to breathe deeply

- Begin to consider the things that drain your energy. Perhaps you have a tendency to overcommit, or find yourself stuck in a relationship or circumstance that no longer serves you. Breathe with each of these places where you feel stuck

- Say to yourself "I have the power to say 'no.'"

- Imagine yourself having the necessary conversation, turning down the opportunity, or simply choosing to remove yourself from the situation

- Feel the power of saying no and being in full control of where you place your energy

- Breathe deeply, cultivating a sense of full peace and security

- Ask yourself "Where are the parts of me that I need to get back?"

- Take notice of every person or place that comes to mind as still having a part of your energy and your essence

- If there are any feelings of melancholy, nostalgia, resentment, shame, or anger, allow them to be there, breathing as they flow through you

- Say to yourself "I release this *person or place*. I reclaim what they have that is rightfully mine."

- Continue to breathe into this empowerment

CPSIA information can be obtained
at www.ICGtesting.com
Printed in the USA
LVHW021736131120
671649LV00010B/807

9 781913 710590